A CLEFT PALATE TEAM
ADDRESSES THE SPEECH CLINICIAN

A Cleft Palate Team
Addresses The Speech Clinician

Edited by

MERVYN L. FALK

Associate Professor and Director
Speech and Hearing Center
Wayne State University
Detroit, Michigan

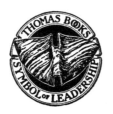

CHARLES C THOMAS • PUBLISHER
Springfield • Illinois • U.S.A.

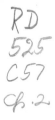

Published and Distributed Throughout the World by
CHARLES C THOMAS • PUBLISHER

BANNERSTONE HOUSE
301-327 East Lawrence Avenue, Springfield, Illinois, U.S.A.

NATCHEZ PLANTATION HOUSE
735 North Atlantic Boulevard, Fort Lauderdale, Florida, U.S.A.

© *1971, by* CHARLES C THOMAS • PUBLISHER
Library of Congress Catalog Card Number: 75-149180

With THOMAS BOOKS *careful attention is given to all details of
manufacturing and design. It is the Publisher's desire to present books
that are satisfactory as to their physical qualities and artistic possibilities
and appropriate for their particular use.* THOMAS BOOKS *will be true
to those laws of quality that assure a good name and good will.*

Printed in the United States of America
CC-11

CONTRIBUTORS

CAROL BARBEITO, M.A.

Formerly, Consultant, Hearing and Speech Section
Bureau of Maternal and Child Health
Michigan Department of Public Health
Detroit, Michigan

JUDITH BENSKY, M.S.W., A.C.S.W.

Formerly, Medical Social Worker
Children's Hospital of Michigan
Detroit, Michigan

ANTHONY R. CERESKO, M.D.

Area Representative, Coordinated Care to Crippled
  Children and Maternal and Child Health
Michigan Department of Health
Detroit, Michigan

NED I. CHALAT, M.D.

Clinical Assistant Professor, Otolaryngology
Wayne State University School of Medicine
Detroit, Michigan

ROBERT CHESKY, M.D.

Formerly, Assistant Medical Director
Outpatient Department
Children's Hospital of Michigan
Detroit, Michigan

MERVYN L. FALK, PH.D.

Associate Professor and Director
Speech and Hearing Center
Wayne State University
Consultant, Cleft Palate Team
Children's Hospital of Michigan
Sinai Hospital of Detroit
Detroit, Michigan

JOSEPH FISCHOFF, M.D.

Chief, Department of Psychiatry
Children's Hospital of Michigan
Detroit, Michigan

E. P. HAWTHORNE, D.D.S.

Assistant Director, Cleft Palate Team
Children's Hospital of Michigan
Detroit, Michigan

J. HILLIARD HICKS, D.D.S.

Director, Orthodontic Department
Children's Hospital of Michigan
Detroit, Michigan

WILLIAM G. McEVITT, M.D.

Chief, Plastic and Reconstructive Surgery
Children's Hospital of Michigan
Detroit, Michigan

K. W. SPROULE, D.D.S., L.D.S.

Director, Department of Dentistry (Retired)
Children's Hospital of Michigan
Detroit, Michigan

PREFACE

IN AUGUST, 1968, a two-week Cleft Palate Institute for school speech clinicians was sponsored by the Wayne State University Speech and Hearing Center and supported with funds made available through P.L. 85-926 by the Michigan State Department of Education.

There were thirty-three participants in attendance who were selected on the basis of geographic location and population density of the area they represented within the state of Michigan.

Presentations were made by members of the Cleft Palate Team from Children's Hospital of Michigan and by representatives of the Michigan Department of Health. Each person's remarks were tape recorded and edited for inclusion in this publication. Comments made to the Institute by representatives of the Michigan Department of Health are included here in order to present a complete portrayal of the integrated information made available to the participants and to provide the reader with a comprehensive view of how one state supports and manages its services to cleft palate children.

One of the more unique characteristics which the reader will recognize is the lack of a prepared manuscript by a speaker. This is readily identifiable by the informal and conversational flavor of each presentation. In order to present a respectable and uncluttered portrayal of the various messages delivered to the Institute participants, some perfecting was necessary at the editorial level. It is hoped, however, that the pages of dialogue which ensue nevertheless impress with their conversational flair. There may even be sentences here and there which seem somewhat disjointed. The only justification for this is that we talk in this fashion.

The reader may also note that from time to time one speaker or another alludes to an issue or makes a point that is somewhat outside his professional life-space. One reason for this may be that the Children's Hospital team has worked together for a long enough period of time that each member has learned a great deal from all other members. The free exchange of information that occurs among team participants and the close professional and personal bonds that mark their relationship complement the acquisition of expertise outside of individual disciplines; this, of course, results in an extra dimension of care for the children who are treated by these team members.

Some speakers, particularly Doctor Sproule and Doctor Hawthorne, used a number of photographic slides to illustrate their presentation. Since it was impossible to include the slides in this book, an attempt was made to refer in the text (as edited) to the cogent features of the films.

I am appreciative of the cooperation of many people who were responsible for the success of the Institute and the subsequent preparation of this publication, namely: Mrs. Susan Greif, Mrs. Olwyn Ballmer, Mrs. Ruth Taylor, Mr. Kenneth Cleveland, Miss Betty Ericksen, Mrs. Lillian Macoule, Miss Glenda Huerta, Mrs. Diane Klemme, and Mrs. Renee Simon.

M.L.F.

CONTENTS

x

Contents

A CLEFT PALATE TEAM
ADDRESSES THE SPEECH CLINICIAN

Chapter 1

THE ROLE OF PUBLIC HEALTH

Anthony R. Ceresko

THE MICHIGAN Crippled Children Commission, as you might be aware, used to be an autonomous agency in the state. Now it is no longer the Michigan Crippled Children Commission; it is the Division of Services to Crippled Children, and it was placed in the Bureau of Maternal and Child Health in the State Department of Public Health for the purpose of co-ordinating preventative and screening services that are provided for in the Bureau.

Carol Barbeito is a member of the Child Division of the Bureau of Maternal and Child Health in the State Department of Public Health. In that manner, total services—comprehensive services—can be more readily administered, rendered, and offered to children who need this type of care in the state. So she is in the Child Division of the Bureau of Maternal and Child Health and I am in the Division of Services to Crippled Children.

However, we are now combining our activities and breaking down into regions, and soon I will be designated as the Area Representative for Coordinated Care to Crippled Children and Maternal and Child Health Services for the greater Detroit area. This will include an area of three counties—Wayne, Monroe, and Washtenaw. The above follows the division of the state into fourteen areas which Governor Romney had requested be followed by all organizations in the state, including ours, the Education Department, Department of Vocational Rehabilitation and the Department of Social Service. I, at present, as I said, am a Medical Coordinator for Services to Crippled Children in the area mentioned above. We are in the process of seeking new office space to accommodate all Maternal and Child Health Services in one office.

As far as crippled children services are concerned, it can best be understood in the manner that I will present it by breaking it down to where our money comes from. First, the Crippled Children Division derives some services from Title XIX. Title XIX supplants former Act 283, that some of you might be familiar with in this state, that provided services for afflicted children. In this program, we provide inpatient hospital care. This provides care for patients who may need hospitalization for pneumonia, appendicitis, or any acute condition, rather than long-term illnesses which require hospitalization according to the judgment of a doctor. We specify only certain hospitals as being able to provide this care and they are actually inspected by our organization over and above the recognition that is provided for by the State Department of Health, Medical Care Division. They judge a hospital purely on the facilities that it has and, to a certain extent, record keeping, and the like, but we go further than that and investigate to what extent they are able to provide care for children specifically, and if we feel that they are able to do so, we approve them for this type of service.

As I said, under this program we provide service for the acute illness that is short term and does not need prolonged hospitalization, or specialized medical care, or does not run into much expense. We permit any licensed doctor of osteopathy or doctor of medicine to provide services in this program. It is important for us to be able to administer the inpatient hospitalization of Title XIX even though by Federal recommendation the program was assigned to the Department of Social Service with payment of services being matched by the Department of Health, Education, and Welfare (HEW). This is unlike Act 283 which used to be totally under our guidance and in which all costs were paid by the state. Federal matching in each state varies and is based on the average per capita income of the people in the state. In Michigan it is practically median insofar as the state provides 50.34 percent matching and the Federal government provides the 49.66 percent. In other states that are poorer, the matching is 75 percent Federal government, 25 percent state government.

The most important area of our activity is our Act 158 program, which is the traditional Crippled Children Act. Funding for this program comes from Children's Bureau which urges that it either be an autonomous agency or in the Department of Public Health and discourages its being placed in the Department of Social service. They match dollar for dollar, to a point, based on a formula of the number of children in the state and giving more credit for children who live in the rural communities. Traditionally in the past, children in rural areas were deprived of medical care. Now, once again, it is recognized that children in rural communities are the ones who are being missed as far as medical care is concerned. Our state quota from Children's Bureau allotment is $1.4 million, and needless to say, our program would require a great deal more than $2.8 million if we gave a fifty–fifty matching basis, dollar for dollar, up to $1.4 million. Our program last year cost $6.2 million, so the state had to provide practically $3.1 million in matching funds to provide care for the crippled children in the state. Now they have revised this. We get $1.4 million from Children's Bureau and match that with state money. Then we go to the Department of Social Service and have the additional money matched dollar for dollar on their basis in conjunction with our total program; but, in order to get this, we have to do special types of interviewing and special types of qualifying people for the program. Some of the employees are totally confused, hospitals are confused, and we are having our difficulties.

Under Act 158, we provide first our field clinic activity. This provides diagnostic service without regard to financial eligibility. You have heard, perhaps, of our field clinics coming into most communities and providing orthopedic, plastic surgery, pediatric, cardiac, or epilepsy clinics. This is primarily for case finding, and it is a manner in which people in the community like yourselves, as well as teachers, public health nurses, or doctors in practice, are able to send children to a special clinic when it comes to a community. This provides expertise in some questionable condition that the child might have, so that it might be determined whether this child may need further follow-up and work-up or that his complaints are negligible and do not need further pursuit. We are now providing this service on an ongoing basis in practically all community areas in the state. We try, in smaller communities or in a smaller county, to combine three or four areas by picking one locale. It could be a hospital or school in the middle of the area, and it is necessary for us to return at regular intervals so the doctors and the teachers and all people who will be referring children to these clinics are able to depend on us. They can expect us to come rather than having a child sent to a specialist in a distant city, if it is possible to wait until the time that the clinic does come to the community. The child can be seen by a specialist in that area and then have further recommendations made from this examination.

When a condition that needs follow-up is determined, there are many dispositions that may be made. The family may be able to pay for its own follow-up care, and a report is sent to the family doctor involved, who makes the decision of the type of follow-up care the child will have. But in cases in which we know that the family might not be able to pay for further evaluation and care, we insert a note stating that we are willing to help the physician develop care for this child by sending him to some center for further evaluation and care. In this manner, we have continuity follow-up so the child is not found with a condition and dropped right at that point.

The specialists who are the consultants for these clinics may be local specialists or, more usually, are brought from the medical schools of the state. They are paid a consultant's fee and travel expenses.

Further, if additional diagnostic rather than therapeutic attention might be necessary for that child, we will pursue it without cost to the family until such time when as much as possible has been done to determine the exact nature of the ailment.

In the past, the clinics used to be a little more haphazard because the communities were not that well organized; but now, with the greater development of health departments throughout the state, we are able to develop greater continuity in the manner described.

Our second phase of activity, and probably more important, is inpatient therapy. This care is provided by a specialist in the particular discipline that is involved with the child. For example, if the patient has cerebral palsy, there may be an orthopedic man or a neurosurgeon involved. If he has a heart condition, he may need a chest surgeon with special training in cardiac surgery and an internist or pediatrician; in this case you may have a team approach. Thus, only specific specialists who are Board certified can provide care under Act 158. Not only does the physician have to be a specialist but also the facility in which he functions has to be approved as having ability to provide such care. Here again, it is our organization that inspects the hospital to determine whether or not this hospital can provide this type of care for this type of specialty.

This, then, provides the basis for quality care under both the Title XIX and Act 158 programs. For example, a patient is admitted with a fever of unknown origin by a general practitioner and in two weeks it is found that he has rheumatic fever. We, as coodinators, can then demand that the doctor have at least a consultation with a specialist or even, in some instances, transfer the patient to another hospital that can provide greater expertise and better facilities. We believe in bringing specialists to a community to render at least a single consultation to see that everything that can be done for the child is being done. We have split our activities in this respect in that we do not stick strictly to the edict of stating that services under Act 158 can be provided only in a 158 facility. In other instances, as in the case of a child who receives a nasty burn and is admitted to the nearest hospital for emergency care, that emergency care can be rendered at that facility, but when it comes to the time when that child may need plastic surgery, skin grafting, and the like, we demand that a plastic surgeon come in on the case. If that particular hospital is not able to provide that care we will have that child transferred to an Act 158 facility, so that both the plastic surgeon and the facilities necessary to provide the plastic surgery are available.

Another aspect of therapeutic care is outpatient services. All children who have certificates of authorization for care under our program are provided outpatient as well as inpatient services. And in either aspect, the care is similarly provided by a specialist, and we provide anything this child might need— braces, appliances, wheelchairs, and adaptive equipment of any kind. For the cystic fibrosis patient, we provide such things as ultrasonic or spray-type nebulizers—whatever might be ordered by the specialist. We buy special beds or special lifts to help the family take care of the child in the home setting. So there is not a thing that goes along with the care of the child that we do not provide. This includes expensive drugs for patients with cystic fibrosis, hemophilia, leukemia, epilepsy, and other conditions. These drug bills might run to $100 and $150 a month, so there should not be any expense to the family. We provide special nursing care for inpatient hospitalization, as well as home oxygen for children who may have severe asthma or an occasional cystic fibrosis patient who needs oxygen at home. Again, I repeat, there is not a thing we do not provide for children under Act 158.

Then, as a special part of our outpatient services, we have what we refer to as special clinics and here is where we come to what we are dealing with today—cleft palate patients. We try to develop special clinics to deal with any condition that may need special expertise. For example, we are in the process of developing hemophilia outpatient clinics at certain locations to which hematologists are being brought. We have our cystic fibrosis clinics at approximately seven hospital locations in the state. We have a nephrosis and renal failure clinic at Children's Hospital here in Detroit. We permit this latter activity at Henry Ford Hospital, Detroit; University Hospital, Ann Arbor; and Butterworth Hospital, Grand Rapids. Thus we utilize what we feel is special expertise to provide a little more than the usual specialty consultation.

To return to the cleft palate patient, we find here a need for combined expertise for the development of the best and most comprehensive planning for the patients. They receive the total care they require, which includes the group consultation and all diagnostic and therapeutic care involved. Here we even leave the hospital to provide such care as pediodontia, prosthodontia, orthodontia, and speech therapy in the community in which the patient resides, to include the doctor's office. We even utilize summer speech camps and programs. There are 1483 cleft palate cases on the State Crippled Children Register.

As an aside, I would like to state that our program is able to provide speech therapy only in two areas; the first is cleft palate and the other is in the area of children with hearing defects, for whom we provide hearing aids. For these latter children, we make sure that these aids are being used properly. We note a study done by Doctor Gaeth * of Wayne State University that demonstrated that only 17 percent of the children that his group were able to examine were using their hearing aids properly at the end of a year. This is a published document. Because of this fact, we decided that we would pay for further indoctrination in the use of the hearing aid.

We were able to do this because our law stated that we were able to pay for indoctrination in the use of this hearing aid for children in areas where this service was not *properly* provided for by the school systems. We use the term "properly" as our interpretative tool and we stepped in and said

---

* Gaeth, John H., and Lounsbury, Evan: Hearing aids and children in elementary schools. *Journal of Speech and Hearing Disorders,* 31: 283-289, 1966.

any child that has a hearing aid can be followed by the audiologic center for any length of time that the Center feels necessary until such time as they feel that both the mother and father are well indoctrinated in the use of this hearing aid so that the child can profit from it. Then, using this as a further interpretation, we pay for the children who were born deaf or nearly deaf, because Doctor Gaeth demonstrated for us that the auditory nerve develops best in the first two years of life and regardless of what is there at birth, if you stimulate this you get better development of the hearing process to some degree. By stimulating this child with a beep so that he might gain from whatever sound does come in, there is some functional improvement, Doctor Gaeth feels, from putting hearing aids on these children who are almost totally deaf. Thus, we provide the speech therapy to help develop optimum potential in this child. So we not only have supported the program here, but there is a similar program at the University of Michigan, one in Mount Pleasant, and one in Flint. We pay for this care of preschool children usually when they are under the age of three or until such time as the child is ready to enter a school program. In this manner, we have entered into a broader usage of the hearing aid. In all of these cases, hearing aids are also purchased.

We feel that there are many disciplines involved in the care of the cleft palate child. What we like to see on a cleft palate team, actually, is a pedodontist (a pediatric dentist), an orthodontist, a prosthodontist, and an oral and/or a plastic surgeon.

In addition, is is necessary to have a pediatrician who will approach the problem with the realization that 33 percent of children with cleft palate will demonstrate other types of congenital deformities or defects and that these should be searched out very carefully.

The team should also include an audiologist, an otologist, a speech pathologist, and a public health nurse. The disciplines mentioned above are basic. However, ideally, it is very desirable to have, in addition, a social worker, a psychologist, and an educator. It is important to have a very interested person in any of the disciplines to assume leadership for best coordination of the group effort.

I will try to show how our program functions in general with hospital clinics. When a child under our program is seen in the clinic, a report is sent to us. When this report is received, copies are sent to the local physician who is involved with the patient and also to the local Health Department. Thus, the Health Department is always aware of what recommendations are made for this child. As I pointed out earlier, the Health Departments are becoming more numerous and better organized in this respect. This means that there will be a continuing effort at greater continuity of care for this child, so whatever might be recommended for this child can be followed through with the local department's help. This is one of their great functions and they cooperate very well in this activity. We find it very gratifying to have them call us and ask us about specific recommendations that were made for certain patients and we are always able to contact the central source of referral for further elaboration of whatever instructions might be unclear to these people and which do not appear on the report itself. Medical coordinators, like myself or our designates, like to be present at the cleft palate conference to interpret our program for its maximal usage. So, there is a constant flow of communication that is developed to provide the continuity necessary for optimal care of the child.

In dealing specifically with the cleft palate program and your part in it, the Health Department can be very active in referrals for speech training, not only to the educational authorities but also to speech pathologists like yourself to provide speech therapy.

This also works conversely. If you have a child who has a cleft palate and who may be in need of speech therapy, you can communicate with the local Health Department to have this child referred to this program. If, at any time, you would like more specific information, you can communicate with the Regional Coordinator involved. In this group, we also include severe maxillofacial deformities. There are five major coordinating regions in the state. This is how we can work together in providing this type of care for these children.

Part of our care for children with cleft palate involves emotional problems that beset these children and their families. I would like to read a few excerpts from a dissertation made by our Public Health nurse who could not be present today; but in any case, I feel that some of the things she mentions here are very poignant as far as understanding the care needed for the cleft palate patient. She said

> Today the habilitation of the child with a cleft palate is more than a surgical procedure. Habilitation must be surgical treatment guided and augmented by medical, dental, orthodontic, and prosthodontic therapy, to promote more normal speech patterns, constant otolaryngologic surveillance, psychological counseling, social and family counseling, plus vocational guidance to explore the individual's potential and to utilize his talents to the utmost.

> It becomes evident that many and varied disciplines must participate in the treatment of the oral cleft child and treatment must begin early in life and continue, possibly, until young adulthood. Since treatment involves many disciplines, it is logical that these various disciplines participate as a unit in the diagnosis, evaluation, long-term frequent planning in order that the patient's physical and emotional needs are met.

> Parental attitudes toward the child rearing and family are important influences in personality development of the child. It is found that mothers with higher education have more approved attitudes toward child rearing. This means that people who aren't too educated, too sophisticated knowledge-wise and can't accept these things must be dealt with even more strictly. And now we know that these children are usually born to younger mothers and, therefore, that brings out the problem to greater relief. And it's more intense a problem in the young mother because she is less apt to accept when others damn. *

Miss Juntti divides the problem into periods of acceptance by the mother rather than of developing rapport by the mother

---

* Juntti, Jeanette: Nurse educator, a cleft palate team member. Unpublished report, Harvard University, 1967.

with the child. The first period, briefly, is a period of deep grief. Secondly, the parents must acknowledge the problem and learn to handle their anger that is involved. Third, the parents must deal with anxieties aroused by the impact of the child's handicap under usual adaptive patterns and then make adjustments in their way of life that will affect not only the child, but the total family unit. Miss Juntti feels strongly that the public health nurse and the public health nurse-educator should play a very important part in the cleft palate team, especially from a point of view of liaison with the hospital so that this type of counseling can start right at the hospital level. She states that "Many mothers are discharged from the hospital with conflicting information from the doctors and nurses with regard to feeding and positioning of the oral cleft infant." And this is true. If you have dealt with this problem, you have found that misinformation is given because of different methods of treatment, or because of ignorance, not considering the infant as an individual. Many parents, because of their attitudes, are unable to cope with the misinformation from professionals during the initial period of grief. The nurse-educator who is scheduling her return hospital visit at feeding time could intelligently work with the mother and other nurses in the hospital regarding the feeding and cleaning of the oral cavity. The nurse, working with the mother, would discover which feeding position and type of nipple are best for the particular infant, thus making the entire feeding process more relaxed and pleasurable for the mother.

You can see that activity for these children is involved on all levels from the time the child is born and then is ongoing. Children's Hospital at present is in the process of developing a psychologist-psychiatrist combination, not only to treat such emotional problems that have already developed in children but also to prevent problems as early as possible by counseling children as early as possible. And we can even go further than that. This has to start with the mother in the hospital at the time of discharge.

Chapter 2

THE ROLE OF A STATE SPEECH AND HEARING CONSULTANT IN CLEFT PALATE MANAGEMENT

CAROL BARBEITO

WHEN I was working in a public school a few years ago, one of my frustrations was that I did not know how I could relate myself to community resources and agencies so that I could make maximum use of these facilities to help enhance the therapy program for the individual child in school.

My current position is with the Hearing and Speech Section of the Bureau of Maternal and Child Health, which is part of the Michigan Department of Public Health. There are ten other hearing and speech consultants working in different areas of the State of Michigan. Each of you in your areas in the state would have such a consultant available if you wanted to gain information about services in your area or to answer questions about a specific child who might benefit by a state-sponsored program.

I would like to relate what my goals are as a consultant to what you might be trying to accomplish in the public schools. Much of my job is helping agencies develop programs in hearing and speech, encouraging good utilization of the resources that are available, and trying to stimulate agencies to work together. Currently, my area is comprised of Detroit, Dearborn, and Monroe County with continued interest in Wayne County, which was my assignment last year. The Hearing and Speech Section is in a transitional stage in developing a complementary working relationship with the Crippled Children's Division of the Bureau of Maternal and Child Health. The former Crippled Children Commission had no speech and hearing consultants on their staff, and problems relating to speech and hearing were delegated to other professionals. Our department, at a state and local level, has begun to attend Crippled Children's clinics representing hearing and speech. At the field clinics held in areas outside of Detroit, our staff provides many of the professional speech and hearing evaluations. The field clinics are composed of a group of professionals viewed as important to the particular disorder. They join together as a diagnostic team for that day and go to a specific area of the state, either to do diagnosis or in some cases to provide care and treatment. The speech and hearing consultants from the other areas of the state have been doing the hearing evaluations and the speech evaluations for all the cleft palate teams sponsored by the Crippled Children Division, and whenever possible, relating their findings to local agencies. In this metropolitan area, the clinics are staffed with speech and hearing professionals. We have two ongoing cleft palate clinics and a number of hospitals which treat cleft palate patients. Sinai Hospital and Children's Hospital are the two major centers that utilize a complete team approach to the problem of cleft palate. I attend these clinics, acting as a liaison person between the Crippled Children Division of the State Public Health Department and the cleft palate team.

The concern of the state would be that a quality, comprehensive evaluation be performed. I think my personal bias in relation to the speech and hearing evaluations is that the cleft palate child deserves whatever would be a good evaluation for any other child in terms of speech and language. By that I mean that he is not just a child who has a hole in the roof of his mouth. His language development, total communication skills, and how he relates to his physical disability are all important. Only when his physical problem has been treated will he be able to communicate freely and use language at a correct level for his age. Until we handle the total aspect of communication in the cleft palate child, we are not doing a complete job.

One of the reasons we are here today is that we had a conference in which clinic people, public health people, and special education people came together. At the conference, it became very clear that cleft palate children need to receive therapy in the public schools, as the clinic programs could never meet the need. The feeling was voiced that the major responsibility for the follow-up therapy and the continuing speech care of cleft palate children rests on the public schools. A public-school speech therapist is able to see a child throughout a long period of his life, rather than sporadically, for diagnosis. Only a limited number of children qualify for and have available clinic therapy versus the number who can be treated in the public schools. Part of the reason for this is that speech, language, and hearing therapy are usually long term and expensive.

Some of the other projects which the State Hearing and Speech Section is currently involved with are based on the conviction that if you do not meet the communication needs of children early and completely, you have an educationally handicapped as well as, perhaps, a physically handicapped individual, and later on you have a work and employment problem. We have been trying to include the infant and preschool population in our programs. We are now doing language and hearing screening programs at the preschool level. Some monitoring of infant communication development is being done. We have emphasized trying to stimulate resources to provide follow-up care for young children. It is a frustrating job to try to build new programs and find the funds to underwrite them. I think this is the same in your school systems many times.

You asked about Title I and Title VI. They are handled through the State Office of Education. At the Maternal and Child Health staff meeting, a speaker came to tell us about the different Acts. Some are very active in the state and others are not. I think there are possibilities for getting these funds for your individual school systems. What you need to do is to demonstrate that there is a group of children who have an unmet educational need and show you can provide a good program for them. Then you write up a proposal and submit it.

I want to mention the cooperative summer camp project between the Crippled Children Division, the Department of Special Education, and the Hearing and Speech Section. This is something that has been very rewarding. There are three summer camp programs in the state for speech- and hearing-handicapped children. There is a program at Shady Trails, which is sponsored by the University of Michigan. They take boys between six and eighteen years. The children have various kinds of speech problems, and of these, only a certain percentage are cleft palate. The cleft palate youngsters are often sent by the Crippled Children Commission to this camp. There is another program at Central Michigan University at Mount Pleasant. This is just for oral clefts. Last year there were twenty-three children sent from various parts of the state to Central Michigan. I think some of these are paid for by the Crippled Children Commission and some are not. Another camp is in the Upper Peninsula, near Marquette at Bay Cliff. This is for handicapped youngsters—malnutritioned, blind, diabetic, epileptic, and those with speech or hearing problems. Special Education pays for part of the Bay Cliff clinic costs and the Crippled Children Commission pays for part. All of these camps are good things. The problem is that the numbers are very limited. However, if you can think of children who would benefit from these summer camps, please let your consultant know. Choose your cases carefully, as there is limited space.

In Wayne County and Detroit, we have been a little frustrated because people say we have facilities. The truth is that our facilities are overloaded and many of them are very expensive. We have been attempting to have some Detroit and Wayne County children included in these summer camp programs. This last year, a couple of children from Detroit went to camp, which was gratifying. If you want a child to attend one of these summer camps, you can contact your local health department or you can call Lansing if you do not know who your regional consultant is. In Lansing, write to the Hearing and Speech Department, Bureau of Maternal and Child Health, 252 Hollister Building, Lansing, Michigan.

The Hearing and Speech Department is not going to be doing therapy in the summer programs, but we are concerned with seeing that the programs are good and will give the child the help he needs. The way we do this is by trying to make sure that the information from the therapists is available to the summer clinic. We work with the public health nurse, the caseworker, or whomever has sent this child through for referral to a summer program.

What is our relationship to you as public school therapists? You may have felt that you wanted another opinion on a child. I think you could usually arrange for the child to attend one of the field clinics in your area for either speech or hearing consultation. At some of them you will have audiologic services, which could provide pure-tone air and bone testing as well as a speech-reception test and a speech-discrimination test. The determination can be made at these clinics whether or not the child needs a full hearing aid evaluation. I think, without exception, that you would be welcome to come and sit in on the field clinics and express the concern you have about a child. You will gain from it and so will the clinic team.

There are other functions that some of you might be familiar with that are provided through our section. One is the hearing conservation programs and follow-up otologic clinic for school children. Most of the counties utilize the hearing conservation programs as established by the Hearing and Speech Section. I have just finished working in a training course for the hearing and speech technicians who do the initial testing in these programs. We have mostly women and only two men technicians in the state. They receive a six-week intensive training course. Four mornings a week they have practical experience in testing children of all ages and mental abilities. This year, we did some preliminary work with screening for language and speech problems in the pre-school child. These technicians have academic training each afternoon and all day Friday. They are usually employed in health department programs. In these programs they first screen hearing at a set level—generally around 20 dB at 1000 Hz, 2000 Hz and 40 dB at 6000 Hz. When the children fail this screening, the technician does a threshold test of hearing. The children's audiograms are then submitted to the County Health Department for review either by one of the county's staff or by one of the state consultants. In the case where the health department has no appropriate staff, the children whose audiograms do not meet standards are invited with their parents to the otology clinics. These are diagnostic clinics funded through the State Health Department. The otologist is present, as well as a public health nurse, the technicians who did the original screening, the parents of the child, and the State Hearing and Speech Consultant. Audiologic test-ing is available at these clinics, which saves the parents an extra trip, as often the otolaryngologist in a private practice does not have an audiologist.

Sometimes the relationship between the hearing conser-vation programs and the speech therapists in the schools is not good and other times it is very good. But I think that when approached with the idea of helping the child both from a public health and education standpoint, information can be gained by working together to help the children. I know in Wayne County we have been glad to have the speech therapist come into the clinics. If they had specific questions, they would come and we would talk it over. I would do what I could to help them and they would bring in children who had other kinds of speech problems and who needed special services. If I could not help, I would try to refer them to other resources.

There is always the question, For what treatment does the state pay? As Dr. Ceresko mentioned, the Crippled Children's Commission has paid for all speech therapy relating to a cleft palate. Hearing-handicapped children can receive funds for the hearing aid evaluation, the aid, and the follow-up training. We have found very poor results from just putting hearing aids on children. They have to have therapy. I think, again, this is one of the frustrations you must have in the public schools because it is difficult to work your hearing-handicapped children into your schedules effectively. Many times you do not have the information you would like to have. This should be available to you. If you do not have it, it might be a good idea to call your health department and try to locate it through your consultant or your local health department. Also you may wish to make another referral to get additional testing for the child.

Once we identify a child at the otology clinic who needs further audiometric evaluation or who appears to need a hearing aid, we will send this child to a Crippled Children's approved center. You will have to ask where your approved centers are. Locally, we use Henry Ford Hospital, Wayne State University, and the University of Michigan Speech Clinic. Preschool children are being seen in a special program in conjunction with Wayne State University and the Crippled Children's Division. The deaf infants range in age from one month to four years.

Further resources are the League for the Handicapped and the Division of Vocational Rehabilitation. I think most of you have a fairly convenient branch available to you. Your health department ought to be able to help you locate it. Both of these agencies are quite interested in hearing and speech problems and in mentally retarded individuals. They will often pay for speech and hearing therapy if you can relate this to the employment of the individual. Twelve-year-olds on up may be acceptable referrals to these agencies.

Chapter 3

PLASTIC SURGERY FOR CLEFT LIP
AND PALATE CHILDREN

WILLIAM G. McEVITT

THE CLEFT PALATE is a cleft in the face and mouth and apparently human beings have been afflicted with this deformity through all civilized ages. They have been observed in Egyptian mummies. On the frontispiece of the book by Doctor Stark, he has a photograph of a head picked up in Peru with a cleft lip. So it is obvious that clefts existed in the pre-Columbian Indian. We must remember that this is a pretty persistent deformity and I suppose it has that in common with all deformities. As you know, it took the human race many, many centuries to increase its population by a rather small percentage, and the infant and child mortality rate was enormous, even in the normal youngster, from diseases and all of the other evil influences. We can be sure that with the added handicap of this deformity, countless thousands of these infants born over the centuries did not survive, but enough survived to carry on. These deformities are very common genetically among us.

As far as we know, the ancient medical works make no reference to any attempt to improve the children, so I would think that you could picture very well the fact in the Roman times, in the Middle Ages, and even in modern Europe through the fifteenth and sixteenth centuries, these individuals must have been wandering around the alleys of Paris and London, and the Italian countryside, completely untouched. This would result in a lot of superstitious ideas on cleft palate. Some of these superstitious ideas were very alive up to the very recent past. I do not hear much about them from the laity anymore but they were very alive even fifteen or twenty years ago. So this thing has been with us all of the time.

What is it? What is a cleft? As you know, the infant's face develops in the womb in sections and these sections come together as the weeks go by to fuse and form the face as we see it in the newborn baby. There are a series of arches, as you know, called branchial arches, and these form the neck and a good part of the face. Sometimes defects of these arches are associated with the cleft of the palate. The face is formed where the central frontal nasal piece and two side pieces called the maxillary pieces come together. They form the face from the level of the eyes down to the level of the mouth angles. The frontonasal process forms the nose and the nasal columella and the central part of the lip called the prolabium, sometimes called the philtrum. This same process behind the lip forms the triangular segment of the anterior palate which is easily identified as the premaxilla. One remembers that it carries the potential of the four upper central front teeth known as the incisors.

The two maxillary processes, one on each side, form the remainder of the palate. If they fail to fuse anywhere, you have a cleft and these can vary from very minimal clefts to any stage and variety of completeness, the most complete being one in which there is no fusion of any kind. Very rarely these are combined with a branchial arch deformity. I asked Doctor Falk to look at an extraordinary child we have in Children's Hospital at the present time in whom there is a total failure of fusion of the left maxillary process and the frontal nasal process resulting in a cleft that not only involves palate and lip but goes up beside the nose to the orbit, or the eye socket, on that side. In addition, the mouth goes way out and there is a deformed ear. I have never before seen these in so extreme a combination and I do not know whether that child will live because it has still another deformity.

Why does this happen? The answer is that we do not know.

Every conceivable type of speculation from the superstitions we have already mentioned have been thought of, and the only thing we are sure of as far as I know today is that there is a genetic element that is very definite. Doctor Fogh-Anderson who practices in Scandinavia and has done an enormous amount of research from a statistical standpoint thinks that some of the clefts, particularly the postalveolar type, are not hereditary but that most of the others are, and he has even calculated odds on what the expectations are. He has written a monograph on this subject. They have a great advantage in Scandinavia. They have a homogeneous population, small and under complete control because of their socialized medicine system, so there is no such thing as people wandering all over as in the United States, on the loose, unreported, or being operated on by people who sometimes know nothing about it. Furthermore, they do not have our mixed population. We have everything, we are getting more mongrelized all the time, and there are hardly any of us except children of immigrants who are pure strains. They do not have that in Scandinavia so they have a controlled laboratory. That is what the country amounts to. If a child is born with a cleft, it must go to an experienced person so they know exactly how many they have, what kind they are, and so on. Working on this, Fogh-Anderson was able to come up with odds for future generations. If you show him a three-generation chart and you show him a cleft somewhere in that line, he can look at that and tell you what the odds are on a cleft appearing in a child which is yet unborn.

Another curious thing along that line is that there is a little town in Holland which is extremely inbred, and for a period of centuries they have had a very high incidence of these clefts—well above average for that country. There are many other causes that have been speculated on. I suppose you have heard of a phenocopy in which you can reproduce a congenital deformity by doing something to pregnant animals like poisoning them or giving them a bad drug or maybe exposing them to x-ray or starving them in various ways. The offspring are deformed. I believe they produce clefts in rats by depriving them of vitamins. And of course there are diseases like German measles that produce various effects. However, no one has demonstrated that any known diseases produce this particular deformity, and furthermore, no one has any evidence that these starvation situations that are produced in the laboratory in experimental animals exist in human beings. Particularly in this country, where we have an excellent diet, we have just as many clefts as anyone else. Furthermore, we could take that a step further. We do not know whether if we did produce this type of starvation in the human being, it would produce clefts. There is no reason to believe that it does because in segments of society under abnormal conditions where there has been terrible starvation, no clefts, at least no more than usual, have occurred.

It is very important for a professional to have fixed in his mind what the mouth looks like. You can study it by looking into a mirror with your own mouth open, sometimes with the the help of a flashlight. Get this thing fixed in your mind. What do I mean to get this fixed in your mind? I do not mean that there is no cleft there. That is too obvious. But fix in your mind the contour of the arch, the thickness and obvious power of those muscles, the thickness and strength of the normal uvula, the position of these pillars in their relationship to the palate as a whole, and the normal depth of the pharyngeal bulge behind the palate. It is quite obvious that a sound mouth and a normal pharynx and the proper movement, and so on, are absolutely necessary to produce normal sounds. Other things are too, but we will not go down below the larynx.

If an individual suffers from being born with these clefts, he obviously has an abnormal anatomic situation and cannot speak normally, and you, of course, know why. In our society, we are usually not dealing with an individual who is in the position of having a totally untouched deformity. But even after the human being has tried to help his brother and repair this cleft, it may still not be satisfactory, and that is the situation with which we deal. When you come to examine a child and his speech is still defective even though his palate has been repaired, you might ask why. Why, after the repair, should the person still have defective speech?

There are many classifications of these clefts and some of them are very complex and really more suited to a study in embryology or some very, very complex sorting system for the few institutions which have maybe thousands of cases on the book. For our purposes, they are not only unnecessary but bad classifications because they are confusing and hard to remember. One classification is that of the late Victor Veau of Paris who did an enormous amount of work, as we shall see later, in this field. He classified them as Types I, II, III, and IV. Type I is postaveolar and a cleft of the soft palate only. Type II is postaveolar also, but the cleft is of the soft palate and extends into the hard palate. The extreme cases have an enormous U-shaped cleft which goes almost up to the teeth. Type III is a complete cleft of the palate.

Sometimes we call the cleft jaw a palatal cleft, or Veau Type IV because there is both a cleft lip and a cleft of the jaw and palate. In other words, the cleft is right through the alveolar ridge and the hard and soft palate.

It is absolutely not true that the bigger the cleft, the poorer the speech. When we get to a discussion of actual surgical operations, we will mention that again, but right here I think you should know that a person can have a cleft and have an operation, even some of the more old-fashioned operations, and when they get to be about six years of age and you examine them, you find they speak normally. Yet you may have someone with a cleft given the same treatment and when you examine them they have a horrible, extreme, nasal escape. The reason is that there are other factors and you should now think back to that normal mouth with its thickness, length, and pharyngeal capacity. It is true that a Type-IV cleft is very much more cleft than any of the others, but in spite of that, if this palate is very short in the anterior-posterior measurement, a perfect repair of this will not give the person normal speech because the palate is too short and they cannot effect velopharyngeal closure.

Another factor is that if the velum is close to normal length but the capacity of the pharynx is abnormally large, once again they cannot make it. Then there is a third factor and this is most important. What kind of muscle does this person have? We go back again to the normal mouth and you remember what you have seen there, what you have looked at, the thickness and power and length of the muscles, because the palate is no different than the human being. You have one man who weighs 260 pounds, has arms and hands like an ape, and has enormous horselike muscles. He may be the star tackle for the Pittsburgh Steelers, or something like that. You see, then, you have another human being who may weigh 115 pounds with very tiny, delicate hands with very thin, light muscles. Palates also vary in this respect and you will see a person with a cleft, and you are about to repair it and you look in the mouth and you see these big thick ridges and these big heavy horselike velar muscles and split uvula but each half looks like a blackjack. Very often an experienced surgeon can look and say this person is going to speak normally or have very little defect no matter what is done as long as it is not a total failure or breakdown.

On the other hand, you come to another individual, let us say they have the same type of cleft as far as the type of anatomy is concerned. You look at that muscle. It looks thin and anemic; the uvula may be a tiny little tag on each side and you wonder about this person. Will he need something else later? You can also get these things in combination. You can have a person with a complete cleft, extremely thin and delicate, with weak-looking muscles, a very short palate, and a capacious pharynx. These differences are very important when it comes time to actually do an operation and select an operation. We are just bringing out the "why" point that the type of cleft alone is not a significant thing in making a successful operation difficult to achieve. These are natural hazards. On top of that, you may have poor results from poor selection of surgery, or a well-selected operation is poorly executed, and so on.

I have made a list of the main reasons for poor results from this second standpoint. We have talked up to now about obvious clefts. There is also what we call a submucous cleft in which there is a true cleft of the palate but the membrane which is visible on opening the mouth either is intact or else has a very tiny cleft of the uvula. The important thing here is that these palates are invariably congenitally short and it is most important for the speech professional to recognize one of these. The obvious cleft is very obvious. Usually you do not see it, anyhow, because by the time it comes to the speech professional it has had some kind of repair. But the children with a submucous cleft traditionally have been discovered late and sometimes never. I have had cases like this that had been in public school or other speech correction classes for years struggling, struggling, struggling to get exercises and to overcome the anatomic deficit they have—which cannot be done. There might be a very rare child who almost made it and if you can build up his muscles he may overcome this, but most of them cannot. Now this situation is changing. We have done so much talking about it and teaching about it and I think here, in at least southern Michigan, the connection between the Wayne State University's Department of Speech and the Cleft Palate Clinic at Children's Hospital has had a great influence on this beccause we have had a number of people trained there to learn these things and of course they come back here. Dr. Falk, particularly, has taught many of these things and his students go out and they begin to pick these things up. The number of these cases to come into surgery now has increased about ten times, I would say, in the last ten years, so it is coming along.

Once again, go back and remember that big, thick palate with the vault and so on. Even though there is no cleft in the uvula, you look in his mouth and recognize the submucous cleft right away because it is thin and short and the pillars do not have the same inclination frequently, and the vault looks too big and you recognize the problem even though the uvula is not cleft. If the child will allow you to put your finger up against that area, you will not hit a normal transverse bone as you do in the normal palate—you will hit some kind of cleft. All these kids most surely would have very defective speech with gross escape and no amount of instruction will help them. In the submucous clefts, the patients cannot achieve closure because the palate is too short and thin, but mostly too short, and the pharynx may be big.

Remember that we talked about the natural handicaps which would prevent people from speaking and then we talked about the bad results following repair which may result in poor speech. I listed the anatomic reasons. The palate is short or immobile. That may be caused by scar, a poorly selected operation, or maybe the palate was so short that no matter what was done it would not be adequate in length. Obviously, there is escape.

Now we will discuss the presence of fistulae. I think the surgeon has to take responsibility for most fistulae. It is very easy to get them. However, I will say that we do not get nearly so many as we did years ago, and that is because we have a wide variety of operative procedures that we can use. The experienced person will pick the safest one for this particular patient. You see, in the old days, and I regret to say, in some places still, they have one way of operating on a palate and everybody gets a fistula. But if you do have a hole, it may seriously interfere with speech. In the clinic, sometimes, one of our ladies or gentlemen will shove a piece of cotton or chewing gum up into the hole and demonstrate an amazing improvement right away.

In another instance, the person may have a successful palate repair in that it does not have any holes and may even be long enough. But if the upper jaw has been crushed in, you have inadequate tongue room and inadequate vault, and you can get a variety of bad speech habits. You will notice that I will not go into these things in detail because you will be taught by people that really know about them.

Finally, I would consider the relation between upper and lower jaw. A bad relationship may be caused by collapse of the upper jaw or it may be caused by an abnormal growth of the lower jaw or mandible; and in the worst cases, you have a combination of both. We will refer to that, also.

Those were the anatomic reasons; so, we went through natural handicaps to successful correction of anatomic defects. Now we have psychological reasons for poor speech. Among them, and these are more self-evident to you, are a low intelligence, an absence of motivation, and hostility. Some people are damned if they will speak well. If a person is always alone, he may not appreciate how he speaks. Maybe the parents speak another language and since they are not with others, others are not noticing that they do not speak well.

Finally, we have the one reason which we hate to admit but which certainly exists. This is where you have a child who seems to have fine muscles, and the result of the surgical repair, so far as you can see, is almost perfect. The palate has excellent anatomy, wonderful contour, seems to move fine, and maybe even when you fluoroscope it, it moves fine and closes but speech is terrible.

To review, we talked about what a cleft is, how long they have been around, what their causes are, and how they are classified, reminding you that there is a submucous cleft. We showed you something about the mere fact that though cleft A is larger than cleft B, A could still be more favorable for the reasons we mentioned. Then we discussed the effect of surgery and the effect of the psyche.

Now we are going to look at the story of man's attempts to repair clefts after centuries during which nothing was done. There is no reference as far as I know in any of the ancient medical literature to attempts to repair these clefts. In fact, there is little or no mention of clefts in the medical literature. An obscure practitioner or barber might very well have done something to repair clefts in the tenth century, but we have no records because of the lack of communication.

The first real information we have about these attempts probably goes back to the sixteenth century and, since the printing press had been invented, things that were done might very well get some circulation. Since those were the days of boiling oil, doctors noticed that a suppurating wound, after it healed to a certain extent, had "proud flesh" (granulation tissue) which tended to stick together. People started putting cauteries on the edges of cleft lips and I am sure that worked. You would cauterize it and scar tissue would form together and you go down farther and cauterize again and that way they probably got some clefts closed. At least they got them together, though probably not the widest ones. I am sure it looked terrible but it was some progress. I think it was the famous Paré who actually closed one by cauterizing the edges and putting a couple of pins across and tying them with strings which actually contributed a force to hold the cauterized edges together. But these procedures were done on lips and no one, as far as we know, tried to close a cleft palate. There are some vague references right at the end of the eighteenth century but nothing really definite.

Very early, in the nineteenth century, surgery was gradually advancing and, within the lifetime of one man, was about to explode. There was a lot of work done in this field. The reason was that the existence of bacteria and infection was not known. There was no anesthesia. Invasion of the abdominal cavity or the chest or the head was impossible because it would always end the same way—with suppuration, infection, and death. As a result of that, a lot of work was done on the relatively superficial parts of the body where you could get away with this. It is an interesting thing that a great deal of work was done not only in this field but in all fields of plastic surgery, which was practically lost to the profession until the earlier years of this century. The reason is that with the advent of anesthesia and the understanding of infection and antisepsis, the surgical profession became fascinated by the possibility of invading the abdominal cavity in curing cancers and finally appendicitis. Other fields of medicine were neglected, including cleft palate surgery.

However, there were always some men who continued to work on it. No one had ever closed a cleft palate. It was thought that if you stripped tissue off a bone, that bone would die, and as a result when they first started with these cleft palates, they didn't attempt to operate on any of the complete clefts but only the number I type in Dr. Veau's classification. What they did was attempt at first to cauterize and then have it stick together. Apparently this worked, at least partially, but the first man to actually get down to business and sew one up was Von Graefe. He just cut the membrane on the surface (he called it peeling) and then he pulled the sides together and put in a row of stitches. He was usually successful, but not always, by any means. Many other people were now doing this and there was a very high percentage of breakdowns and failure. The reason, we know now, is that by just peeling the membrane off, they had a relatively thin piece of tissue with a poor blood supply. Another German surgeon by the name of Diefenbach finally succeeded in closing a cleft by the method of peeling off the membrane and sewing it together.

Simultaneously, this was being experimented with by other people in other parts of the world who had no idea that the same thing was being done elsewhere and one place was here in the United States in Boston. Doctor Jonathan Warren did the same thing as Diefenbach did, although there were a lot of breakdowns and the procedure was very unsatisfactory. Then a man who may be the most famous name in cleft palate surgery, Bernard Von Langenbeck, while working on a person with a cancer of the roof of the mouth, noted that in removing the cancer he had stripped the bone bare, and though he expected it to die and slough, it did not. He had been doing some cleft palate work, so he reasoned that if the bone did not die, why not go after one of these palates and instead of peeling the membrane go right down to the bone and take the whole soft-tissue covering off the bone, including the periosteal layer of the bone. The procedure is called a mucoperiosteal flap. The bone did not die and immediately the percentage of success went up. They were doing comparatively few because they did not have anesthesia and they would give the person a lot of narcotics and put ice on it attempting to numb it. It must have been a terrible ordeal and I am sure they had a lot of deaths, and so on. But, anyway, it was successful. That operation ever since has been known as the Von Langenbeck operation. Probably more repairs have been done by that method in the last one hundred years than by all other methods put together. It is still in use by some people.

Other people—we won't go into the detailed history— advocated various types of relaxation incisions of all kinds, even cutting the tonsillar pillars because they were getting into the well-known problem. As long as the patient had a very narrow cleft, the surgeon could lift up the mucoperiosteum and sew it together. But when the cleft got very wide, this was under such tension that once again they were breaking down. So they came along with all these methods of cutting the sutured muscles and this helped, but often it was at the expense of good function because sometimes they would cut very important muscles.

This operation went on and people in other countries learned to do it and it was no longer, especially with the advent of anesthesia, unusual to close cleft palates in children. The mortality was still high—often 10 or 15 percent died. From 1861 down into the later part of the century there wasn't too much change.

There were some other rather bizarre operations suggested, one of them by Sir William Arbuthnot Lane in England, but they really never took hold. Then, toward the end of the century, people started to realize a certain fact which brought the world eventually into a second phase. They realized that, in spite of successful closure in many cases, the speech was terrible. People started studying this, mostly in France. One of the earliest was a Doctor Passavant in France. He under- stood this problem and he tried to do something about it. He tried sewing the back of the soft palate against the back of the throat. He tried putting in mechanical devices, too, because he realized it was due to disproportion between the length of the palate and the pharyngeal situation that they could not get velopharyngeal closure. He first of all described the bulge of the pharynx coming forward to form a ring with the posterior palate to effect closure and it has since been known as Passavant's pad. I think you know where that is. He then tried filling that. This is a big step forward because it recognized that simple anatomical closure often failed.

Then, another Frenchman by the name of Victor Veau, the same man whose classification we saw before, began to study this very carefully. He concluded it was wrong to cut these muscles, and he realized that a soft, movable palate was important. He came along with a very important contribution. Instead of cutting the muscles, after he had dissected the palate off the bone, he then went superiorly to the nasal side and dissected tissue off the upper surface to the bone. He could then stretch it out and put in a double layer of sutures. First he sewed together the nasal-membrane side and then he sewed the mouth side together so he had a perfectly lined palate which was longer, and he did not have granulations or contractions. The speech results were better because we have a longer palate which was more capable of reaching back and closing. He also had a lined palate which did not suffer from postoperative contracture. This was a very important consideration. Doctor Veau was very active in the early years of this century.

A number of other European surgeons visited there; one of them was the late Professor Kilner of Oxford University. As a young man, he spent more time in Paris with Doctor Veau than he did in London. He told me an enormous amount about him, which was important because he later made great contributions himself. The contributions of these French people were noted and they helped him a lot. There was still a lot of nasal escape present, however, from all accounts.

The action now goes back into Germany where a doctor by the name of Ganza, in thinking about this thing, applied a certain technique used in other parts of the body to make a piece of tissue longer. This is well known. Supposing I go in and I make a V-shaped cut. Having cut through, I can now slide the two side pieces down to the center piece. We will lengthen our original V, and it is longer and what letter is this? Hence the V-Y. That has been used in many innumerable patterns worked out for various tissue parts by what we would call plastic surgery today. But Ganza applied this to the palate. What he did was to cut in such a way that if you projected his two lines you get a V. Then he cut it off the bone and pushed it back so that the point moved posteriorly. His uvula had come together and he now has a Y. And the palate is longer. As far as I know that was the first trick like that done and it was quite good. Others followed. Then came the English, e.g. Wardill and Kilner. Because they were studying these patterns and also patterns of others, they were making many trips to Paris and together they decided that if you used a pattern like this and combined it with Doctor Veau's dissection of the nasal membrane, so you would not have contractions, you would get a long, soft, lined palate that would be the longest ever. And they went farther; they adapted this to a complete cleft. You notice this has three flaps. They adapted this to a complete cleft by fashioning four flaps. This was an enormous advance and they worked this out in the mid-1920's after World War I.

As far as I know, there was not a single such procedure being done in the United States at the time, and if anybody had heard about it, they certainly did not confide in me because I was taught to do the Von Langenbeck operation in a classical manner. Later, when I was in Detroit, the late Doctor Straith, who did almost all the work around here, did what was basically a Von Langenbeck operation, but he buttered it up with a cutting and suturing of the posterior pillars of the tonsils together and wiring the front of the cleft. This was very traumatic and the results were often extremely poor. He learned this from the late Doctor Brophy in Chicago. He, to the best of my knowledge, never changed the technique as long as he lived. In any case, in addition to my being taught, I used to do a lot of traveling in those days and I saw these palates being repaired in cities like Baltimore, Philadelphia, San Francisco, Chicago—all Von Langenbeck. At Hopkins they did a classical Von Langenbeck operation using heavy black silk sutures. Von Langenbeck could have done it himself. This was as late as 1940.

Meanwhile, in England, they were doing V-Y four flaps by the hundreds and getting excellent results. I was in Detroit at this time. I was desperately struggling to improve results and here, at this point, we might say I have never seen any method of repair, no matter how illogical it may seem or no matter how crude or how old, that did not sometimes produce an excellent result. This, of course, produced much confusion. Remember what we talked about earlier—about thick muscles and long palates. If you had such a case that had such excellent potential or maybe superior potential, it seemed no matter what you did to it, as long as it was not a complete breakdown, you would often get a good result. I will not mention names, but I remember one doctor who, when he had a good result, always called people in to hear the excellent speech. But he never called in anybody to hear the one that was still nasal.

I first saw the V-Y done after I had been struggling like crazy here in Detroit because I finally realized that after examining hundreds of children we had only this occasional person with an excellent result. I remember one person—a young man who had his palate all chewed up and could sing almost a high C. He fancied himself operatic material. I was trying to do two things. One, I was trying to sew the top of the palate—I will not go into this in detail—farther back hoping to reduce the size of the opening that was to be closed. The other thing I was trying to do was to dissect the nasal membrane, as Veau did, only cut it way back so that when it slid back there would be no raw place on the movable part of the palate. About this time I had my first opportunity to have a conversation with Professor Kilner. This conversation lasted about an hour and a half and I learned more from him in that period than I learned from all the American surgeons that I had talked to in a number of years before. It was a wonderful opportunity because you did not have to explain anything to him. The minute you talked about what you were doing and what your problem was, and so on, he understood it more completely than you did. With my technique of cutting the membrane way forward and then sliding it back, he said that he had done that for a while and he said it was a perfectly logical thing to do but it is unnecessary since you get as good a result by stretching. Later I had an opportunity of watching him actually do a palate. By this time I was doing V-Y four flaps though I had never seen anyone do it. But after I saw him do one, I did it 100 percent better. He had done a matter of fifteen hundred of them by the time I saw him. This made an enormous improvement in speech.

For years now at Children's Hospital, as Doctor Falk can testify, we have children who come up to the clinic who have had this done who speak normally. Now we know that all of them do not, but there is a number who just speak normally. We ask, "Is the speech normal?" The answer is yes. There is another very large group who have relatively minor defects who work out with the ordinary instruction and who speak normally by the time they are nine or ten.

However, you have the number who do not speak normally and you have to find out why. This brought the whole thing to a rather high level. Then the third phase was entered because we found out that some who have long, soft palates were still nasal and everybody had them and that other things must come into the picture—a lot of other things. At first you know nothing and you tackle the most obvious thing which was to close the cleft—just get it closed. Then you get more critical and you attack the problem of why the closed cleft still produces poor speech. We started asking such things as why the speech is poor. The palate is closed. It seems to be long. In this case, it may not be long enough. Can it be lengthened further? The jaws are collapsed and there is no tongue room and maybe articulation problems are severe.

Do not forget that picture of the mouth. Let us assume that we are bringing a child in here and this child is five or six years of age. Let us also assume she was born with a cleft palate and it was repaired sometime in the past. We would now undertake to talk to the child and examine the child, trying to make an appraisal of her condition. In so doing, there are many things we might encounter and these things would include just about everything that you have had as either a question expressed or in your mind. First of all, What would the ideal situation be? The ideal situation would be that the child had a cleft, had reasonably good muscles, reasonably good length, all the things we talked about earlier, and that she was operated on by an experienced operator who took these important factors into consideration— such as lining, length, and so on. As a result of this, this little girl speaks normally. That is a delightful result. If she speaks normally, there is nothing else for us to do. I do not know what percentage of our own children speak normally. I do not think we have ever gone back in the records and figured that. Probably we should do that some day.

On the other hand, everything under the sun may be wrong with the child at the other end of the spectrum. For years and years this sort of examination was managed solo by the surgeon who did the operation. He would listen to the speech, look at the child's teeth, and so on. If it looked good he was very proud of it and if it did not he did not do much about it. Meanwhile, in another sector of the city, there would be some poor conscientious dentist who had a person who had no roof to their mouth and horrible speech. It was just driving him so crazy—he was trying to correct this with some sort of prosthesis. Maybe on the floor above, there would be a nose-and-throat specialist struggling with a totally deaf child or nearly deaf child. Out in the public schools, there was a poor girl who had started with high ideals, who had a little boy that was just about unintelligible and she had beaten her head against the wall, scolded him, and everything, but was not getting very far. Twenty-five or thirty years ago here there was one doctor who was doing most of the work. If the speech was fine, he would demonstrate it. If it was not, he would tell the parents the same thing. He told them two things. One was that there is a very fine speech department in the Detroit schools, which I think was true but not very helpful to the mother. The other was that he recommended that she get a book, the title of which was *Sounds for Little Folks*. Between *Sounds* and the knowledge that there was a great speech department in the public schools, the mother went home to struggle with this child who was close to being unintelligible. No real analysis was made as to why the child was unintelligible; or if there was something you could do; or, if it was possible for this poor girl in the famous speech department to get anywhere at all; or, was she under an impossible handicap? The conscientious people of the world have been trying to do things like that.

Our first attempt at other help here was when I decided I would keep a record of all of the children I contacted, chronologically, in the order of their birth. I entered their names in this huge book which was spread on the table. We would put type of cleft and something about their history and their progress along the line. When a report would come in from the school or from a dentist or from a nose-and-throat person, it would be entered into that book and that way we had some kind of a running record. Also, this chronological record would tell us whether a child had been in for a check-up or not. Supposing we would want to look at something after a two-year interval, say in 1952. We would go back to the 1950 list, just turning the pages back, and it would tell us right away whether they had been in. This helped a whole lot. Most of the people I was dealing with were the people that I knew very well and were also interested. I can remember Doctor Hicks and I having luncheon and discussing this subject twenty-five years ago. Finally we decided that we would be more efficient if we started meeting in a group. There were some other groups operating in the United States. It was really a tremendous improvement because we had all of this very experienced talent there at the same time looking at the same child and we did not have any correspondence back and forth or phone calls or anything. We could do it then. You had to learn how to do it by doing it.

Our weakest section was speech when we began. We could not seem to get any qualified people or to keep them. That was later wonderfully corrected. When we look at a child, we have a nose-and-throat specialist and this is very important because these children, if they are neglected, will get ear infections and become deaf. They need to be treated and sometimes operated on by a nose-and-throat specialist. Doctor Chalat will go into that with you in detail. We have the speech and hearing. We test the child's hearing. We then make an examination of its speech, and this is, of course, the thing you are more interested in than anything else.

If we had that one little situation which I described a few minutes ago, we can just be pleased and that is the end of it. But that is not always the case. We have cases that do not always turn out well. Sometimes we see some terribly chewed up children who have been worked on elsewhere. Let us take the speech. Remember the reasons for poor speech we discussed before. Let us start from the back of the throat. If this child has air escaping, this is one of the most serious things. The first thing we do is make a clinical evaluation and x-ray examination to see if the palate, as it is, is long enough and movable enough so that this child could achieve good speech. If the answer is yes then the appropriate therapy is recommended. Suppose the answer is no. Almost always the reason is that the palate is too short. It may also be immobile. For a long time we had experimented with various methods of secondary lengthening of those palates, and we found out that it was also true of the submucous clefts, that we were not successful, no harm had been done, and the child would need a pharyngeal flap. We short-circuited this situation and if that is the case, the pharyngeal flap is recommended and done. We have had a high percentage of success. The younger it is done, other things being equal, the better the immediate result. We have some outstanding cases. We did a pharyngeal flap and by playing the preoperative and postoperative tapes, we found that the person converted to normal speech—but we do not expect that ordinarily.

However, the usual postoperative analysis by a speech professional is that the improvement is very definite and the situation is such that with some training as to how to use the flap, normal speech will be achieved. Supposing the palate seems to be long enough but there is a hole in it. We will, if we can, close that hole, and usually I would say that 90 percent of them can be closed. If for any reason it is impossible—too big, too chewed up from previous work—then we may go to the dentist for help to put some kind of cover over that.

While we are talking about the dentist, suppose the jaw is crowded and has poor tongue movement. The orthodontist comes along and he will expand that. In so doing he might produce a fistula. In other words, it has been crowded together, and as you can see, when the jaw is put in a normal position, there is a space in there and that would have to be closed. In some instances it might have to have a bone graft. Finally, if the jaws are in excellent position, there may be some other difficulty because there are teeth missing. Then the prosthodonist comes along and fixes that with either a fixed or removable appliance.

Among your questions has been that concerning a child who has a rigid palate who escapes and whose speech is poor. Without seeing him, you can be sure his palate is either short or immobile, or both, and if we examine him and determine that he could not achieve normality through therapy, he would get a pharyngeal flap. That is what would be done to him.

I thought you would be interested to hear about some of the other work we have done. One of the big problems in these things is this collapse problem, and it is a very serious problem. It narrows the jaw, it may interfere with speech, it produces very bad dental malocclusion, it gives inadequate support to the lip and nose and so it is a cosmetic liability, a dental liability, and a speech liability. For about sixteen years, we have been slaving to try to do something about this and we think we have discovered something very interesting. Back in the mid-1950's in Europe, they started doing a lot of bone grafts, particularly in Scandinavia, and then a Scotsman by the name of McNeil did them, in these collapsed and maloccluded jaws in quite young children of two or three years of age. They started putting acrylic plates in their mouth and fixing them with a dental adhesive. The jaw was out of position and the plate was maybe a few percentage points closer to normality than the jaw. In a young child like that, two or three years of age, what was happening was that the jaw would be forced to accommodate to this plate and in so doing would move somewhat toward normality. Then this wily Scotsman would make another plate which was still closer. In that way, he would tease this thing along and the next thing you knew, he had it in normal position. Then, the idea in many places was to try to hold this by bone grafting it. Since you can not do everything, we had a different dream which was in the newborn baby with a gap in the palate. If we could only hold that, then maybe it would remain normal.

The idea at first was to bone graft that gap, and we would take the bone graft off the pelvis of this little baby and wire it across the gap—but it did not work. The power of the repaired lip is so powerful that it pulled it together anyway into crossbite or some sort of malocclusion. Next we tried carving a piece of hard silicone plastic and wiring it in there. That did some good but it was not good enough. Then came pourable silastic and we were now able to pour on a model a plastic appliance which snaps up in the baby's mouth and fills up the whole cleft so that the cleft cannot collapse. What we wanted to do was hold this thing in position until the baby was six months, a year, or a year and one-half old, and then bone graft it. We actually did some bone grafting.

Then one day while reviewing one of the models, we found something which was quite surprising to us. The appliance was not made so it went all the way up to the front of the cleft because we were afraid it would impinge upon tooth buds and on the lip repair, so we left a little bit open there. To our amazement, with a succession of models taken two or three months apart, the tissue on each side of the cleft in front of the appliance was growing into the front of the cleft. By the time the youngster was eight to twelve months of age, it had grown in all the way and it was solid. This means that if you had a big wide cleft and the appliance fills it up to about here, since the appliance has that thing plugged, it can not collapse. Then this side can grow out and this starts to grow out, so that by the time that kid is nine months old this is no longer a complete cleft. It is a postalveolar cleft. It has converted Veau's Class III to Veau's Class II. This is most interesting. Strangely enough, it makes the technique of closing this cleft more difficult because in a big wide one you do not get the advantage of collapse. As a result, you have to know all kinds of tricks to close it, because in former times, with every method, this would come together in front and this would be much narrower in front and a little easier to close. So we made ourselves a problem in so doing. I think this is very excellent. We are in the process of getting ready to report this and it is a long, complicated article which we have been working on.

In any event, this is the way we look a youngster over today. We analyze them by specialty. I do not know if anybody else does it this way because most clinics will have a certain number of children come to them and they will bring a youngster in before the panel. The child feels just like he is in front of the *Gestapo*, you see, and then they will select certain ones to discuss. We started off by doing that, but we abandoned it very quickly and we switched over. It was in 1956, twelve years ago. We put each child in a separate room with the parents, and then all these members of the panel, different specialists, visit each one of the children. So it is the child's own bailiwick. He is the host. There is a lot of difference between sitting in a room with your mother and father and having people coming in and visit you and sitting there with a couple of armed guards behind you and bright lights on you—quite a difference. We will take a group of about six. After everyone has seen the child, we will have a meeting and discuss each one, not certain ones, but each child, and get the opinion of each specialist, and of course they can talk back and forth with one another. This is very important, because sometimes, for example, something Doctor Falk does not know Doctor Hicks might be able to tell him. When we get the compound opinion, the recommendations are made and those are taken back to the parents and provision made for activating them.

Chapter 4

OTOLARYNGOLOGIC PROBLEMS OF CLEFT PALATE CHILDREN AND THEIR MANAGEMENT

Ned I. Chalat

I KNOW THAT most of you people here today are primarily concerned with speech. I am primarily interested in hearing. But I do not believe one can talk much about speech without having at least some interest in hearing and in knowing exactly how the two are related. Interestingly, the problem of the cleft palate deals with both speech and hearing because the cleft palate child has a great amount of hearing loss. The earliest papers on cleft palate children and cleft palate surgery considered speech and hearing deficiencies to be related. This assertion is borne out by our figures, which indicate that between 86 and 90 percent of children who have a cleft palate problem do, in fact, have either hearing problems or ear infections, or both.

I think the team approach to cleft palate treatment is extremely important. So important, in fact, that I feel I should discuss it at length. Let me say at the outset that confusion exists for the parent who is confronted with this multidiscipline problem unless there is some way of organizing treatment. It is discouraging for the mother to go to various doctors only to find that there are innumerable problems, many of which cannot be handled all at once. If there is no program set up for the child, it is obvious that both the patient and the physician will suffer.

The first mention of the team approach was in 1930. I suppose you know that in that year, one of the early years of the Roosevelt regime, the Social Security Act was recommended. At that time it was believed the Act would include medical benefits. Probably the Blue Cross was what forestalled its advent until just recently. But the White House Conference in 1930 considered bringing unrelated specialists into groups for the advantage of the handicapped child. The disadvantages of rigid specialization and the inability to communicate problems and ideas were evident even at that time. In the Social Security Act of 1935, although medical benefits were not provided, it mentioned a cleft palate program, and stimulated by the Act, Doctor Cooper organized in 1938 in Lancaster, Pennsylvania, the first known cleft palate team in the United States. In 1946, a team was developed at the University of Illinois under the Division of Services for Crippled Children. The team immediately noticed all of the inadequacies in the previous methods of handling these children.

The idea of the group, of course, is that participants may endeavor to treat the child as a whole rather than concentrating on their own individual specialties. The aim should be to study and to apply all available knowledge to the growth and development of the patient. The participants of the group must be willing to use the team approach to this very complex problem.

Basic to the team approach is that each team should strive toward maximum efficiency, possess adequate physical facilities, and secure consultation wherever indicated. Further, according to Harkins, an ideal team should include a team leader, preferably a plastic surgeon because he is perhaps basically responsible for the ultimate outcome of the child; a prosthodontist, an orthodontist, and a pedodontist. At Children's, we happen to have each. In addition, there should be a pediatrician, speech therapists, psychologists, an otolaryngologist, a social caseworker, and a vocational counselor. I personally feel that we should also have an audiologist. The audiologist in our clinic has been invaluable because he frees the otolaryngologist from conducting hearing tests, which enables the latter to concentrate on the physical treatment of the child. Obviously, secretaries and nurses are also needed.

I would like to say, too, that in my original paper on this topic, I suggested that the pediatrician and the psychologist need not be in constant attendance. I have come to find that this is a mistake. By excusing the psychologist and the psychiatrist from early attendance, we have faced some really serious psychological problems with some of the children. In retrospect, it would have been far wiser for us to include this man in our original clinic, and we would have had, hopefully, fewer problems than we do now. The object of the clinic, of course, is to provide children with a closed palate with good speech, not good speech for a cleft palate child but good speech for a normal individual—one who is cosmetically acceptable and who can also fit normally and happily into our society, fulfilling all of the functions of the student and adult.

QUESTION: Is getting these people together expensive?

ANSWER: It is not expensive. I contribute my time—many of us do. I think that rather than expense you should consider creating interest. If the interest is there people will come. Obviously there is a job to be done here. In terms of expense, if that is a real problem, I know that facilities are available through the Rehabilitation Office and through the Federal government. We know, too, that many of these patients can pay a certain amount each visit with the new Michigan Variable Fee Schedule of Blue Cross and Blue Shield.

QUESTION: What is the incidence of cleft palate?

ANSWER: This is a comparatively rare congenital anomaly. In Denmark, where they have a system of socialized medicine and can do calculations and statistical studies on genetic relationship, they found that the incidence was one in 665 births. The incidence seems to be gradually increasing through the years. And it is slightly higher than the one in 800 live births that is generally the figure quoted in the United States. Speaking of the genetics, Doctor Fogh-Anderson's studies indicate that if two apparently normal parents have a cleft lip or cleft palate child, the risk of recurrence is down to about 5 percent, so that you need not recommend against having children if this has happened once in the parents' experience. If one parent has a cleft lip, the chance of deformity is about 2 percent in their children. But if a deformed child has already been born, the chances rise to about 15 percent in subsequent children; that is, if a parent with a cleft palate or lip has a clefted child, perhaps about 15 percent of their subsequent children may expect to have deformity. In general, we feel that patients should be advised against marriage if both partners have a cleft, especially if it is of the same genetic character.

Doctor Emanual Skolnik, in his article "The Otologic Evaluation of Cleft Palate Patients," (I'll quote the source because it is a classic) * evaluated the function and the purpose of the otolaryngologist in the cleft palate team. A review of this work is really unnecessary, I think. We should emphasize at this point, however, that the important factor is regular attendance by the otolaryngologist. If he appears sporadically or if he is not present for many of the meetings, enough patients slip through in a short period of time so that his value is really minimal.

The first thing we have to do, of course, is take a careful history. The history should include hearing loss, presence of ear infection, and mouth breathing as it relates to both nasal deformity and the hypertrophy of adenoids and tonsils.

If you are interested in the questionnaire approach, there was an article in the *Laryngoscope* of June, 1968, by Doctor Maxine Bennett of the University of Wisconsin, who presented a paper which included a cleft-palate–oriented questionnaire about children. It included some of the questions that

---

* This article appeared in *Laryngoscope, 68:*1908-49, 1958.

I have already mentioned—the presence or absence of hearing loss, a careful description of speech as it may relate to hearing loss, age, and when and where the cleft palate surgery was performed, because it is known that surgery by different doctors, even in the same community, will have different results. Information on the following points is also very important: allergies, general health, other birth defects, the presence or absence of other diseases which may affect hearing, such as measles, mumps, meningitis, jaundice, and scarlet fever; and the presence or absence of drugs which have been given to the patient, such as neomycin, quinine, streptomycin, and kanamycin. All these factors must be considered in history taking.

The physical examination is also very important. I think that no matter who you are or what you are doing, it would be advantageous to you and to your patients if you regularly examined the ears, for you can then detect the presence or absence of wax, infection, or pus. Almost anyone can do this. If wax is present, it is really a waste of time to do much hearing testing. The presence of wax means conductive hearing loss and most of these children we are discussing have problems with conductive hearing loss. Whether it is actually disease or wax may not be known, but it would not be known unless you looked. Hearing testing is tremendously important, though. Since most of you do your own hearing testing, you know the difference between conductive and nerve types of hearing loss. If the bone conduction is better that the air conduction, the probability is that this is a conductive hearing loss. If they are the same or if there is a falling-off curve, you will know that there is nerve deafness.

In the series that we evaluated here, I think there were about 3 patients out of 325 who had nerve deafness. There were two patients who had lop ears and two who had complete atresia of the external auditory canal—obviously a severe conductive deafness. There was a large group of other related congenital abnormalities—about 19.8 percent. Actually 20 percent of the youngsters who had cleft palate or cleft lip had related congenital anomalies. I can run through these. The highest percentages involved clubfoot (I am not aware of any specific syndrome, but it is interesting that clubfoot would be that high a percentage); some children had nasal deformities; micrognathia, which would be the Pierre Robin syndrome, accounted for six children; and there were four youngsters who were believed to be mentally retarded; two were bleeders; two had congenital heart disease; two had lop ears; two actually had congenital laryngeal defects; and three had nerve deafness. That is an important factor. Categorically, it would be a mistake to conclude that everybody who has a hearing loss with cleft palate must also have a conductive loss.

One of the important points I want to make is the obvious advantage for research which accrues through the team approach. I became involved in this area very early. Perhaps I should tell you a little more about my own relationship with the clinic. When I came back from the Air Force, it seemed that at about the same time as I was entering private practice Doctor McEvitt was starting the cleft palate clinic at Children's. At that time I volunteered to spend one day a month with the youngsters. It soon became obvious that there was a great need here because, as I mentioned earlier, a large number of these children were hard of hearing. It was also evident that the biggest problem in hearing was related to their recurring ear infections. If the normal child comes in with recurring ear infections, the first thing one usually recommends is a tonsillectomy and adenoidectomy (T&A). And, of course, I was immediately confronted with the problem of whether it would be wise to recommend these procedures. The first thing one does when he is unsure about what to do is to review and evaluate the literature to determine what others have thought about the problem.

I should now, therefore, like to review some of this literature just to show you how ambiguous it can be and also to show you how people who rely too much on clinical judgment can make serious mistakes. Literature regarding the advisability of tonsillectomy and adenoid surgery on the cleft palate patient varies from "always" to "never." None of the articles had questioned the desirability of clearing up the infections of the nose and throat. However, most of the objections to surgery were similar to Doctor Gibb's, who preferred not to do tonsil and adenoid surgery because of the risk of hypernasality in the child's speech. On the other hand Doctor Joseph Sataloff reviewed 30 patients from five to sixteen years of age, and he referred, too, to the conclusions of other doctors. Of the 30 patients, 29 had pathology of the ears. Only ten gave no history of frank ear infections. He recommended an adenoidectomy in every patient who was diagnosed as having a cleft of the palate. Those are the first two articles I read.

Doctor J. Daniel Subtelny quoted another physician, Doctor Calnan, who warns that there is risk of permanent nasal speech following adenoidectomy. After reviewing the physiology of the palate and adenoidal mass, Doctor Subtelny concluded that since we cannot preoperatively predict the adequacy of closure of the palate, conservative management and lateral adenoidectomy are indicated. Doctors Halfond and Ballanger write that the prime factor in hearing loss of the cleft palate child is middle-ear pathology. That is obvious. They reviewed 69 selected cleft palate children; 32 of them were without hearing loss. They concluded that the tonsils were the primary factor in this pathology, but they admitted they did not know the exact relationship, but they assumed that the tonsils were the focus of infection for middle ear infection and eustachian tube dysfunction. It is their belief that the importance of the tonsils in speech production is much less than the importance of insuring adequate auditory acuity for speech perception. Doctor Halfond believes that the risk to speech perception through retention of the tonsils is greater than the mechanical threat to speech production. In other words, he is in favor of tonsillectomy. He did not mention adenoids in his paper.

Doctor Hugh Gibson Beatty wrote that no child should

be denied the removal of obstructed or infected pharyngeal lymphoid tissue. However, he describes a special operation in which he retains a strip of the posterior tonsil and capsule. These are then sewn together with the posterior pillars. The effect is to close further and then lengthen the palate. This surgical procedure was actually done long before he mentioned it, but he revised the previously described technique. This procedure has proved to be ineffective and has fallen into disrepute. This is because though the palate is lengthened posteriorly, and although the oral airway space may be shortened, it is not effectively pushed back far enough. Doctor Skolnik, whom I have already mentioned, did a very comprehensive study of about 400 cases at the University of Illinois. He found that 45 percent of the patients had ear pathology, and of these 39 percent had hearing loss. He found an interesting age differential. Only 21 percent of the children under one to four years old had ear infection, while in the five- to thirteen-year age group, 69 percent had ear pathology. Ear disease was present in 53 percent of the cases with good closure of the palate and in 79 percent of the cases with short or inadequate closure. In other words, if they had a short palate, they were more likely to have ear pathology. He concluded that the age of the child at surgical repair did not affect the percentage. However, it would seem logical to assume that if one could effect a good closure in the one- to four-year age group, the percentage of ear infections would be cut down. He mentioned earlier in his paper that only 21 percent of the children up to four might have ear problems. I think that even though he did not project it into his paper, the age of closure is important. In fact, we are closing the palates at a younger and younger age. Doctor Skolnik found only 32 percent of normal ears by thirteen years of age. He also found in his study that 84 percent of those children with enlarged tonsils and adenoids had ear pathology, while a considerably smaller percentage of children with small tonsils and small adenoids had difficulty with the ears.

There are several other articles, but I am not going to

quote them, except the one by Doctors Masters, Bingham, and Robinson. These gentlemen drew three conclusions which I think are significant. (a) Audiometrically detectable hearing loss secondary to congenital cleft of the palate is an important and as yet unsolved problem. (b) The former goals of cleft palate therapy, particularly in normal speech and normal facial growth, must be enlarged to include normal hearing if the rehabilitation program for children is to be adequate. (c) The high incidence of hearing loss in the cleft palate appears to depend upon the type of defect. Although I have not mentioned it before, several other papers have alluded to this fact. If a patient has a bilateral cleft, he is almost certain to have ear trouble. If he has a cleft on the right side (which is less frequent than the cleft on the left side), he is less likely to have ear trouble than trouble of any other kind. The left-sided clefts have about 50 percent ear infections. The lowest incidence of conductive deafness occurred in those who had lengthening of the palate, while the highest incidence of deafness occurred in those with a prosthetically repaired cleft. In their series, Doctors Masters, Bingham, and Robinson expected that 80-plus percent of the patients that had prosthetically treated clefts would end up with ear infection. This has not been our experience with the new prosthesis that we are using here prior to lip repair.

To summarize what I found by studying the literature, Doctors Gibb, Berner, and Calnan were opposed categorically to tonsil and adenoid surgery. Doctors Halfond, Ballenger, Skolnik, Holmes, Reed, and Sataloff were very much in favor of tonsillectomy. Doctors Subtelny, Beatty, Masters, Bingham, and Robinson all suggested modified surgical procedure. There I was. I had just as many for as against and some who suggested a different operation. Nobody had actually taken a group of children to see what does happen if you do a tonsillectomy and adenoidectomy. So we devised a project in our clinic. While reviewing the literature, it became apparent that no one had ever done a number of tonsil and adenoid operations on cleft palate children and then evaluated their results, both on speech and on hearing. The histories and hearing of the cleft palate patients at the clinic were carefully evaluated and the cleft of the palate was not considered a contraindication to surgery.

A series of cases were undertaken. At the time of writing this paper, 38 children had had their hearing tested and 51 children had had their speech evaluated both preoperatively and postoperatively. This was done because some of the children had severe ear infections toward the end of the series—severe enough so that we were not able to test their hearing at that time, but we did conduct good speech evaluations. I admit that these particular operations were done with great care and perhaps more than usual attention was given toward preservation of the palatal and pharyngeal musculature. Hemostasis was, wherever possible, obtained by pressure. Ligatures and ties were used very deliberately and discreetly, although this was very difficult to evaluate. No sclerosing solutions were utilized. Incidentally, it is the habit of some physicians to use Monsell's solution or silver nitrate as a chemical cautery to control bleeding at the time of surgery. This procedure was avoided. All of the available lymphoid tissue was removed; that is, both adenoids and tonsils. The hearing had been uniformly tested on a recently calibrated Allison-MA-1 audiometer. The project was carried out in 1962, so the hearing loss was recorded in decibels as per A.S.A. standards. The loss was considered to be the average threshold at 500, 1000, and 2000 cycles per second. Of the youngsters that we eventually operated on, 83 percent of them had unilateral clefts. As in all statistical studies, there was a preponderance of males.

Let us look at the results. In evaluating the first-visit hearing loss, we took 96 of the children that had not had tonsillectomy and adenoidectomy and evaluated their hearing. Their hearing loss for a uniform group which we thought did not have and did not need tonsillectomy and adenoidectomy at the first visit was 12.7 decibels. After we did tonsillectomy and adenoidectomy on the post-T & A group, their hearing loss was 3.4 decibels. That is well within normal range. Then we evaluated the speech. Again, we had 38 patients on whom we did tonsillectomy and adenoidectomy and we found that the speech was improved. For those who had undergone tonsillectomy and adenoidectomy, the speech was carefully evaluated by the parents, by the speech pathologist at the clinic, and by me. Thirty-one percent of the children were reported to have had improved speech. We did not actually expect anybody to have improved speech after this operation. We considered the possibility of its worsening. Thus we had to speculate on why the patient's speech was better following a tonsillectomy than it was before surgery. For one thing, we thought that the improvement was due primarily to the reduced nasal obstruction caused by the adenoid mass. We also noticed that the tonsils in some of these children were very redundant. Since they were down in the back of the throat, we felt they might possibly have interfered with the motility of the tongue. We therefore concluded that less nasal obstruction and better motility and mobility of the palatal muscles and the tongue were the reasons for the improvement. Of the children, the speech of 63 percent remained the same, which was really very gratifying. That meant that a total of 94 percent had the same or better speech. The speech worsened in three children on whom we used this procedure. It turned out that each of these youngsters had a special problem. One had a cleft that had not been operated on. He had been seen at the ear, nose, and throat clinic where it was determined that he needed a tonsillectomy and adenoidectomy. The parents were unaware of the cleft of the palate. We did the T & A. His speech got worse; then it got better again after the palate was repaired. The two other children had very bad speech to begin with. Congenitally, they had very short palates that could not be adequately repaired. They were both candidates for a superiorly based pharyngeal flap. So we not only knew they had speech problems but we anticipated further palatal surgery before the T & A. This was gratifying. It was as important to me because I felt that I could now do a T & A in good conscience on a youngster that I felt might need it. The paper was important because we presented it at several national meetings where it was well accepted. Further, it was important because it showed the potential for research in a group such as this. Though it is probably not the final answer. Doctor Bennett of Wisconsin showed that she can get almost the same results by sectioning the levator veli palatini. She did a research study on some 53 patients in which she sectioned the levator tendon as it came around the hamular process and she felt that this, as it affects the eustachian tube, was a factor in infections. Now this just reviews again the speech problems.

That was just another example of a research project. Another interesting observation was made when we were doing a great deal of preoperative testing on children with conductive hearing loss. At that time we discovered, or we thought we discovered (again we got into the situation where we found that someone had described it first), that in youngsters with a conductive hearing loss the bone conduction would move up if the fluid was present. We used this knowledge, then, for a diagnostic study. This one research project evolved into another research project. So we still had a great deal of interest in the middle ear and exactly what happens to the hearing when fluid is present and when there is conductive hearing loss as a result of secretory otitis.

QUESTION: How recently did you present this?

ANSWER: I presented it in 1964. As a matter of fact, I got another request for a reprint about a week ago. I presented it at the American Laryngological, Otological, and Triological Society. It was also presented at the American Speech and Hearing Association by Doctor Evan Lounsbury, and at the American Cleft Palate Association meeting in Mexico City some time ago.

Let us talk more during this hour about some of the basic otologic approaches and the problems that we encounter. I am first going to talk about the mechanism of the conductive deafness which occurs. Now why do these youngsters get into trouble? Obviously there has to be something about this congenital abnormality that predisposes to ear infection. What is it? It is not as obvious as we originally thought. The middle-ear space is filled with air, as is the external auditory canal. We have known for a long time that the problem with the middle ear is the Eustachian tube, that there is some malfunction of this tube. In many children, it causes ear infection to become a disease of childhood. The ear naturally makes a secretion just the same way as the mouth makes saliva and the nose makes mucus. This secretion, probably a mucus, drips down the eustachian tube into the back of the throat and is swallowed with the rest of the saliva.

We believe that is some cases, for some reason, dysfunction of this tube is simply due to the hypertrophy of the adenoids. For instance, we know that every time we swallow, the tensor opens the eustachian tube and permits air to enter. We are also aware that in a youngster who has a large adenoid mass, breathing through the nose is completely obstructed; consequently, drainage of the fluid can be stopped with the result that the fluid tends to accumulate in the middle-ear space. This in itself is dangerous for three reasons. First, this fluid is a great medium for germ growth, so these young people who have fluid in the ear have recurrent ear infection. Second, the fluid, if it remains in the ear for some time, becomes very thick and sticky. So if you hear the expression "a glue ear," it is because this fluid, after remaining there for awhile, actually has the consistency of glue. It is a thick, yellow substance which obstructs sound. Third, adhesions then form and permanently affect the ear. Furthermore, there have been recent theories that chronic otitis media with perforations of the eardrum can result from this fluid because these adhesions drag in particles of tympanic membrane which create a cystic mass that we call a cholesteatoma. It is also dangerous because the presence of this fluid very often affects the hearing, and I feel that hearing on a day-to-day basis, particularly of a child, is important. This fact is especially significant in our very competitive society. If a child can hear today and not tomorrow, he is in trouble because he gets himself constantly involved in situations with which he cannot cope. "Today I can hear well so I'll sit in the back seat." The next day, because the eustachian tubes are not functioning, his ears are filled with fluid so he does not hear well. But he does not know this. Perhaps we can compare it with wearing glasses—you do not know what you are missing unless you have your glasses on. Thus, unaware that he is not hearing as well as he did yesterday, he will get in the back of the room and do badly. If you question these parents over a period of time you will find that suddenly these children are not doing well in school. Obviously, the major factor here is the presence of the fluid in the ear, and removing the fluid is important. Basically, doing a myringotomy, a lancing of the ear, and aspirating the fluid so that air is replaced in the middle ear space is the objective you wish to accomplish.

One of our aims should be not only to treat what presents itself but to prevent its recurrence—preventative medicine. Therefore, when we find that a child has repeated episodes of ear infection, that upon examination he has a thick, tenacious fluid in the ear, and that there is a history of trouble over a period of time, we believe we should not only remove the fluid but do whatever else is possible to prevent its recurrence. It is at this point that the adenoids and the tonsils enter the picture, because anything that can obstruct and create bacterial infection in the nose and throat can be a factor in this problem. Basically, what actually happens is that when the youngster comes to the office with the first episode of trouble, I may recommend a myringotomy. In fact, I may recommend two successive myringotomies. Should these procedures fail, then we would recommend the tonsillectomy and adenoidectomy. So I do not routinely do a T & A on every child with hearing loss. His particular problem has to fit into certain categories. Again, I feel that the adenoids are primarily at fault. The proximity of the adenoid tissue to the eustachian tube cannot be overlooked. On the other hand, my own experience indicates that when we take out the adenoids and leave the tonsils in, we encounter some future problem with these children. Consequently, this means a second anesthetic and a second operation for something that we might easily have accomplished at first. So unless there is some other reason such as allergy, or the parents or the pediatrician are specifically opposed to a tonsillectomy along with an adenoidectomy, we usually recommend a T & A, since our purpose is to cure the patient. This one-time approach is considered best.

There is one other point I would like to mention here. Recurring ear infection in children runs in families. I do not believe this is hereditary. But just as people in families tend to look alike, I do believe that whatever the dysfunction of the eustachian tube is that makes a child predisposed to this condition, it is present in family groups. I can use the example of my own family. My wife, for instance, had recurring ear infections as a child; she actually had a mastoidectomy when we used to do that operation for ear infections. And my daughter (who fortunately favors my wife in looks) had a great number of ear infections until she had a tonsillectomy and adenoidectomy when she was about six. Personally, I have never had an earache in my life and my son, who favors me, has never had an ear infection. I think that if we consider this problem on this basis, because people will come in with one, two and three children in the family who all have this sort of trouble, and you explain it to them as I have done to you (through the facial features concept), they should then understand that it is not a usual hereditary problem.

I promised that I would talk further about secretory otitis. We believe it has been a significant problem since the advent of the antibiotic era. Very little literature exists on this disease prior to discovery of antibiotics, probably because every time fluid accumulated in the ear there was bacterial infection and this infection was the real *bête noire* written into the otolaryngologic writing. You are all familiar with the fact that until some years ago, at least when I was a youngster, the threat of acute mastoiditis for children was great. Here in Detroit at Harper Hospital there was usually one mastoidectomy a day. One of the physicians who practiced at Harper at that time had an assistant, an immigrant physician who on Mondays, Wednesdays, and Fridays went to the west side of Detroit to change only mastoid dressings, and on Tuesdays, Thursdays, and Saturdays did the same thing on the east side. At Children's Hospital here in Michigan, an average of three mastoidectomies per day were done during the pre-antibiotic era. Naturally, nobody would want to go back to that time; I am not advocating that as a happy period even for an otologic surgeon. The objective of a physician is to stamp out disease. Fortunately, with our shortage of doctors, we no longer have to face that critical problem. But we are more aware of other problems that can lead to secretory otitis, a disease which hampers hearing and reduces the performance of people in society.

This fluid that accumulates in the ear is one of the problem factors in children. "What do you do about fluid in the middle ear space?" is the question asked in almost every ear, nose, and throat journal published today. I have prepared a slide on this subject to show some of the complexities involved in handling this situation. First, diagnosis of the presence of this fluid is not easy. Every time I do a T & A on a youngster, it is my practice to take my binocular illuminated operating microscope and focus it in on the eardrum to see if there is fluid in the ear. Frankly, I am not always certain. Neither am I always certain whether fluid is present when I examine the ear in my office. The fluid, as it initially forms, is the color of saliva. Those of you who have examined the tympanic membrane know that the eardrum normally has a greyish or practically translucent color. I liken the normal ear drum to looking through an old-fashioned bathroom window. We are not exactly sure about the pathologic mechanisms creating this disease. Neither are we certain whether it is an abnormal formation of a fluid, a mechanical malfunction of the eustachian tube, or an allergic condition in which allergy affects the opening of the tube. I also want to point out that we are not even sure about the hearing problems that arise in patients with secretory otitis. There is certainly a lack of uniformity of accepted treatment, and whenever you find different ways of handling a particular problem you know there is no one adequate treatment. Further, the prognosis is unpredictable. If a patient comes to me with a child that has this problem, I tell him about 85 percent of the youngsters that have a myringotomy with removal of the fluid, together with adenoidectomy and tonsillectomy, have no more trouble. This is an accurate figure. But there is the remaining 15 percent who have persistent trouble. For reasons that are not too clear to us, the incidence of this disease has increased over the past several years and frankly, we do not know how to prevent this problem. It may be impossible to prevent the recurrence of this fluid in some individuals.

An associated fact discovered when we were doing hearing tests on children suffering from this disease was that very often the bone-conduction test would be up to –10 or –20 decibels, which is as high as we could test on the audiometer. At that time I was working with Doctor Evan Lounsbury, an audiologist, and he postulated that hearing was actually better than –10 decibels. So we began doing some hearing testing along that line. We simply removed the filters that interpolate between air and bone conduction recordings and tested hearing at better than –10 and –20 decibels by bone conduction. The result, we found, was that when fluid is present, we would get an air-bone gap in spite of the fact that the hearing may be almost normal.

I am now going to discuss just such a case. This is the case of a four-year old youngster who came to the office with apparent fluid in the ear and definite thickening in the eardrum. His audiogram showed an air-bone gap. In fact, his hearing loss in his right ear would probably not have been picked up by a school audiometer. We did a myringotomy and aspirated the fluid. These are interpreted by I.S.O., the standard of measurement since 1964. Later, the child returned again with fluid in the ear despite the myringotomy. We again found this sort of an air-bone gap. We removed the fluid and inserted polyethylene buttons and his hearing was found to be normal.

The idea of a polyethylene button or tube is to replace a malfunctioning eustachian tube. If an infection is present, the eardrum will usually burst by itself, breaking in the weakest part of the eardrum. If we deliberately make an opening into the eardrum by lancing it, we can make the opening on a part that usually heals well, namely in the posterior-inferior aspect of the ear drum. There is in this area of the eardrum four discrete layers—an outer epithelium, an inner epithelium, and a radial and a circumferential layer of connective tissue so this will heal well. Where we lance an ear in this area so that it will open up is just one of the problems. Not infrequently, the myringotomy or the incision will heal before all the fluid has come out, and this is a situation we have to face. That is why we try to aspirate and draw as much of the fluid as we can at the time of surgery. Putting in a plastic polyethylene button or strut provides a permanent opening in the eardrum. These devices usually remain in place by themselves for about three to six months and are then thrown off by the eardrum as the epithelium heals behind it. We reason, therefore, that this procedure enables the ear to rest for about six months. This slide demonstrates the hearing possible with the tube in place. Take the tube out and the fluid comes back. Again, normal hearing on a pure-tone audiogram is a little better by bone conduction.

QUESTION: Do you have an awful lot of trouble with keeping the tubes in the children's ears? It would seem that if they cough real hard, blow their noses real hard, or during sleep, that they could come out quite easily.

ANSWER: They do come out—I would not say too easily, but they do come out. I would like them to stay in as long as possible. At the symposium we had in Miami recently, one of the participants, discussing this same problem, said that he managed to keep a tube in an eardrum for about fifteen years. Actually, I did not know that many people were doing this procedure that long ago. There is a tube described that actually has a metal clip on it which goes around the malleus. If you want to leave it for a long time, you should hook the clip to the bone. I had trouble in getting it in one youngster. As a matter of fact, I put this tube in a grown-up and it came out anyway. Fortunately, most of them stay in for about three months and then come out by themselves.

This is the final result in the child just mentioned. We reinserted the tube, kept it in for about six months and then took it out. The mother was in the other day with another child in the family that has the same problem again and said that the first child has not had more difficulty. He had to have that tube in a total of nine months before he apparently grew out of the trouble. The object of these remarks is to tell you that it is difficult to make a diagnosis of this problem and to emphasize that we have to rely tremendously on the audiography. Sometimes special testing is required to verify the presence of fluid.

There are various types of polyethylene tubing. Usually the youngster has to be asleep in order to insert it. When we talk about it falling out, it does not actually clatter out into the bed as some of the parents expect it to do. It just falls into the ear canal and can be easily removed in the office. I have never myself seen a permanent perforation of the eardrum following the use of this procedure. On the other hand, it is more common to have a recurrence of the problem. Obviously, three months is a very arbitrary figure. It is simply that that is about how long it takes before the tube falls out by itself. In preparing my paper on this project, I found that of the thirty-eight tubes that I had inserted in the two-year period during which I had conducted the study, only three children were clearly well after we had taken out the tubes. They, then, are three children that probably would not have been well if we had not used this procedure. Of the total of thirty-eight children, all were well while the tubes were in place. However, we have done nothing about the basic disease by putting this polyethylene tube in for a while. The object of this treatment is to deliver the child to adolescence when he normally grows out of this problem and enjoys healthy ears and good hearing. Failure has to be looked at rather stoically. What I mean is that if we do something for the child and it has not worked, we just have to either repeat what appears to have been the most effective treatment or go on to something else.

All of this is not talked about purely as an infection. As I said, some of these children will get actual, literal germ infection. The symptoms of this are not simply hearing loss. Symptoms with bacterial infection in the ear now become fever, pain, and drainage from the ear. If this fluid becomes infected, you have these symptoms added to the stuffy feeling and loss of hearing. This problem has now to be treated even more seriously and treated with antibiotics. I need not go into this treatment because it really concerns medical management, but basically it involves antibiotics to kill the germs.

As far as you people are concerned, the most important aspect to remember is that adequate follow-up is necessary until the ear is completely well. The number of mastoidectomies for chronic infection that we do at the medical center hospitals today has been increasing ever since the advent of antibiotics and we believe this is due to one of two things. It is either an infection by coincidence or an organism or germ that is resistant to the antibiotic, and we are finding that to be an increasing problem today. On the other hand, it may also be due to the fact that the child develops pain and fever and is then treated with an antibiotic, so the symptoms disappear. In other words, symptomatically the child seems quite well. Thus the parents, and possibly the physician, consider the child to be well and do not really examine the ear carefully or obtain hearing tests to make sure that the hearing has returned to normal. The result is that infection persists, scar tissue can form, and chronic otitis and mastoid infection may follow. The next infection would almost assuredly be associated with a hole in the eardrum.

Chronic bacterial infection must be considered seriously. It is leading to most of our problems today which involve radical ear surgery. At one time we could only operate on the ear to eradicate infection. Since World War II, our knowledge of the physiology of the ear has increased so much that we are able to do mastoid surgery that can have as its goal not only the creation of a dry, noninfected ear, but the restoration of hearing as well. With these two attainable goals, we are able to operate on more people than formerly and our results are infinitely better.

I promised I would talk about the feelings of one particular author on the value of parents. I really do not know. Personally, I believe that you can believe parents when they come in. If you cannot believe the patient who has the disease, or if you cannot believe the parent whose child is affected, who are you going to believe? Even in cases of compensation, I am inclined to believe what the patient tells me. On the other hand, a positive history of ear disease in approximately 50 percent of the cases was all that was found in a series conducted at the University of Wisconsin. These results did not always correlate with the otologic abnormalities noted. Parents, generally, could recall serious illness but tended to consider their children average or very healthful. Positive or negative history of past disease in the Wisconsin series was found to be of little value; that is, in trying to correlate the history given by the parents on these exact forms with the actual physical and audiologic findings of the children. I really did not get that involved myself.

One of the important things you should know is that if there is bacterial infection of the ear, a culture and sensitivity study should be recommended if early antibiotic treatment has not been effective. It is possible to take a specimen of pus or germs from the ear and send it to a clinical laboratory where they can grow the germ and study it with the various antibiotics. This is known as a sensitivity study. Through this test-tube approach, a direction is given for further antibiotic therapy. This test can cost anywhere from seven to twenty dollars and is usually paid by Blue Cross or by the majority of insurance policies in effect today. The wide-ranging antibiotics normally cost from thirty-five to fifty-five cents a capsule. It is less costly to be more scientific in cases where you find the particular antibiotic, and administer it in high doses, that is going to kill a specific germ. One time we did a series at the hospital when we tried to evaluate just what organism created an ear infection. We could not tell. We could not tell by the odor and we could not tell by the drainage. Neither could we tell by the history of the infection nor by the proximity to other people with other infections. We could not tell, either, which antibiotic would be most effective. Just as soon as I suspected that the youngster had a staphylococcus infection, it proved to be a yeast infection. Using other than a scientific approach should be discouraged.

Allergy is a big predisposing factor in terms of ear infection. And there is some relationship between allergy and the tonsils and adenoids that is not clearly understood. I have had in my own experience three youngsters with asthma who were cured after the tonsils and adenoids were removed. As these were rather specific cases, we suspected, even before surgery, that they might be allergic to the bacterial allergy. Each time they got a cold, their doctor termed it asthmatic bronchitis. Unfortunately, and more commonly, the child who has a predisposition to allergy will have a worsening of symptoms after the tonsils and adenoids have been removed. We are not clear about the cause. It may simply be that the youngsters were allergic to the pollen and dust in the air. Because of the large adenoid mass, the air could not get in and out of the nose. So it was their breathing air into the shock organ of the nose that created the allergic symptoms. At least this is one possibility. There may be other factors as well. At any rate, we are a little more reluctant to remove the tonsils in children who have an allergy than we are to remove the adenoids. So if you encounter a child with recurring secretory otitis, make sure that you check him for the possibility of allergy.

Diabetes can create recurring infections. The blood sugar is high. We did a locus-menora-resistentia, an area of low resistance in the body which may well be the ear. This will be the infected area every time the diabetes goes out of control. Another condition is called hypogammaglobulin anemia in which the gamma globulins which control the immune response in the blood are not adequate. This again is an hereditary disease and has to be considered in patients who get frequently recurring infection. Hypothyroidism and other debilitating diseases such as tuberculosis and leukemia generally can reduce the resistance of a patient. Anemia is another factor. It has been my experience to treat youngsters who have frequently recurring ear infections and recurring throat trouble. We take them into the hospital and usually find their blood hemoglobin is not high enough to risk an anesthetic, so we send them home. By the time we get their hemoglobin back up, an operation is unnecessary—they are well. These are some of the things that should really be looked into and considered before the day of surgery.

I want to talk now about some of the other factors that we meet which are not directly related to cleft palate children but which we see in these youngsters anyway. They are the necessity for diagnosis of nerve deafness, the requirements for hearing aids, and the way in which we select hearing aids for the patient. Another problem involves vocal nodules because not infrequently we see singer's nodes in these youngsters as well as in other children. I would like to tell you how I feel about this problem. For one thing, I have come to believe that the singer's node is a disease of the young American male. As a matter of fact, I was at a meeting in Chicago where Doctor Brodnitz spoke. He deals primarily with the voice problems of the actor and singer in New York. It is his contention that it is strictly a disease of the middle-class American youngster. He thinks it is somehow related to little-league baseball. Actually, this is not necessarily true. Personally, I think it may be due to camp in the summer time. At any rate, it is a disease related to vocal abuse. The singer's nodes we are talking about are vocal nodules. Diagnosis is usually hoarseness and generally occurs in the seven- to nine year-old age group. The disease is progressive. Typically, it becomes worse in the summer and is most severe when the child comes home from camp.

QUESTION: Concerning papilloma . . . ?

ANSWER: Papilloma is a different disease. It is essentially a wart on the vocal cord. A true papilloma under the microscope is pathologically a different disease. Singer's nodes or nodules are just hyperkeratosis—just a thickening of the skin. They are more like a callous or a corn. Papilloma is probably a virus disease, like a wart.

It should be clear that the nodule does occur in young women, too. And it occurs in grown-ups as well. I think I may be a candidate although I have never had them. If you listen critically to the voice of the patient that has this problem, it is a little higher pitched than one would expect his voice might be. It is due in part to a combination of vocal abuse, by screaming and hollering under a tense situation, and to poor speech habits. There was a time that once we had made this diagnosis, we would suggest surgery for these youngsters; that is, surgical removal. However, I have grown away from this approach. Although I still remove them in certain individuals, I feel that at least a period of voice training ahead of time is indicated. When I see these children in my office because of severe hoarseness in summer and fall, I usually recommend that, if possible, they secure help from you people in school—help to reeducate their voices to try and take away the strain from the throat and bring it down into the abdomen. Now this is difficult. I know I need not tell you people this, but the speech habits begin at about two years old, and by the time we are seven, they are so ingrained that it is often very difficult to reeducate them. I think that whatever can be done is important.

If nothing else, you can get the youngster to know the importance of being quiet. A vicious circle develops because these children who have this hoarse voice, if they yell, Hey, throw me the ball in a ball game, are probably going to get it because the other players can tell who yelled, whereas the other youngsters whose voices may be somewhat similar and less distinctive will not be as effective if they call for the ball. So one of the things I tell them at the outset is not too much "hubba-hubba" when they are playing baseball. They can be the quiet ones. Hopefully, this sort of exercise will begin to make the nodules disappear. They do not disappear overnight any more than the minute you take off a bad pair of shoes you get rid of your corns. It takes a long time for them to disappear. So, I reevaluate the youngsters myself around Thanksgiving to Christmas time to get some impression again about the way they sound. I also talk to the parents critically to see if they feel there is improvement, and if necessary and possible, I get in touch with the speech teacher to see if the youngsters are making any progress with the voice. If they are, I will temporize—try to put the surgery off for some time. If there is obviously a worsening of the condition, I suggest an anesthetic and removal of the vocal cord nodules. Ideally, we would like the youngsters, adults, or whoever we do the surgery on to be quiet for a couple of weeks so that the vocal cords can regrow. However, we are getting into some emotional problems in this area. It is very difficult to have any person quiet for two weeks and then expect them to go back to talking without being sort of wound up in the way they sound. So I am increasingly less critical of the parents and more and more inclined to tell them that their child may soon be able to go back to whatever talking may be essential, and not to make a big emotional thing about not talking after surgery. I have perhaps come here hoping for some suggestions from you people about this emotional problem because it is a real one and we see very many children with it. And I am moving gradually away from unnecessary surgery; yet on the other hand I have seen some fine results from careful surgery. Obviously the surgical approach without an attempt at reeducating the voice pattern is, I think, worthless and should be contraindicated.

QUESTION: About the Pierre Robin syndrome . . . ?

ANSWER: It is micrognathia along with cleft of the palate; small jaw related to the cleft of the palate. Because of the small jaw, youngsters with this problem have either an apparent hypertrophy or an enlargement of the tongue. And they have a lot of trouble breathing immediately after birth. I do not know if you see these patients when they are terribly young, but you should certainly be knowledgeable about the problem. A significant percentage of these children have Pierre Robin syndrome. Six of those in my study (six of the forty-five that had related diseases) had Pierre Robin syndrome, or micrognathia, along with the cleft palate. It seems to me I recall another figure in a recent article. At any rate it is significant—six of forty-five other related abnormalities. The problem arises of how a young or a newborn baby manages the large tongue—manages to eat with an already clefted palate, for very often they get into trouble. They will be slow to gain weight, quick to aspirate, and unable to manage the nipple or even the gavage feedings. We have come to learn that in these children, the best treatment is a tracheotomy. In spite of their young age and the possibility for other abnormalities, the tracheotomy will enable them to breathe while they are eating. In one case, it was necessary for us to leave the tracheotomy tube in for eighteen months following birth before we could remove it. Generally speaking, the normal growth of the jaw and repair of the palate will outdistance the large tongue as a problem and then you can remove the tube. But if you find youngsters with this syndrome that I have just described doing badly and who seem to be having a great deal of trouble breathing, you should call the problem to the attention of the doctors and, if you can, suggest they should know how to do a tracheotomy. Other things have been recommended, such as sewing the tongue to the lower lip, but these are not generally considered to be as effective.

QUESTION: How do you solve the problem of the cleft palate youngster when he is born . . . generally try to send him to an area where there is a clinic?

ANSWER: Some people, in spite of the fact that transportation is what it is today, are not able to do that. Personally, I think that in areas where there is not a standard team setup it would be a good idea to organize a consultation or a confrontation with the various doctors involved in the problem, even at a local level. You do not need to have an organization meeting every month; I think it is an advantage, obviously, because the quantity of patients is an advantage to the physician who is training and handling the problem. On the other hand, if you do have patients who cannot avail themselves of the clinics that are at hand, you should at least do what you can on a local level to get the appropriate people together around a table to talk about the youngster. Otherwise, the situation is quite hopeless. I am sure you are aware of the parent who has to see all of these people and is not given some instruction or help in seeing to it that it can all be done and meshed into his financial potential. It could be a real problem. There is no question that the team approach is important; we are now expanding this type of approach to other problems. The hard-of-hearing child himself, who is born with a hearing loss and who has a hearing loss at a young age, obviously can benefit from the same type of approach; speech teachers, speech educators, hearing-aid people, otolaryngologists, classroom teachers. It is a more limited approach, but still the same group of different disciplines approaching a problem do better if they can talk it over themselves and present a uniform group of suggestions for the patient.

I thought I would talk to you about hearing aids. How many of you deal with hearing aids and hearing testing? For those of you who are already dealing with them, there is perhaps not much I can say. We believe that the younger you can get hearing into a youngster, the better off he is. Ideally, if children can hear sound and be aware of sound at the age that they should be learning speech, you can teach them speech more handily. On the other hand, we are crowding the area in which we cannot test them with cortical audiography, with the EEG audiography, which is currently in a little more disrepute than it has been. But with various types of tests, we are approaching the ability to test at the age that the child needs the aid. There have been several papers written recently that imply that amplification may further damage a youngster's hearing, and so this factor has to be considered seriously. I personally am not sure myself just which side of the fence is correct. We know that noise damages the nerve of hearing; we know that people who are involved with noise have a tendency to lose their hearing more rapidly. However, we know we must get noise into these youngsters if we expect them to function properly. So here we have a problem which we are going to have to face again. It would be better if we could do research in large enough quantities to get the answer to this problem, and soon.

Hearing aids will only amplify, of course, what the youngster is able to hear. It is obvious that the child who wears a hearing aid well is going to hear well. In general, the air-conduction aid is better than the bone-conduction aid. And certain youngsters with atresias, or with atresias along with congenital cleft of the palate, will, of course, do better with a bone-conduction aid. Unless there is enough ear canal to insert an air-conduction receiver, or even if there is no eardrum, they may do better with the bone aid. It is difficult to fit these youngsters with hearing aids. Again, I am an enthusiast for some such facilities as we have here in Detroit—The Rehabilitation Institute, the University, Ford Hospital, and certain private offices in which there is equipment to test the children carefully and to select different aids that would be adequate, rather than simply recommend them directly to a hearing aid salesman and thus lose some control of the situation.

Now you all know that the state has a program for screening youngsters in order to isolate hearing problems, and probably many of you are very active in it. In 1960 and 1961, we evaluated what happened to some of these youngsters who were tested. During that time, 420,000 children were tested in the school systems with pure-tone audiography. These children were divided into counties and cities. Of these youngsters, a percentage had a permanent hearing loss, a nerve deafness, and they were not particularly referred to hearing people or to otologists. Some of them who had previous knowledge of ear disease were seeing a doctor. A total of 8,634 children were recommended to see their doctor to seek more help regarding their hearing loss. In following up this group, we found that not all of them went to their doctor to seek help. But the results were very gratifying. Of the children who went to their doctors, seventy-seven percent had their hearing restored, or had improved-to-normal hearing. I would say that is a pretty good batting average. Twenty-two percent had either a greater loss or their hearing had not improved. Of these, 50 percent, or in other words half of the people who went to see their doctor about these problems, had normal hearing when they were tested the next year; 27 percent more had improved hearing.

These are the figures for those who did not follow medical advice. This is the percentage of children with hearing loss diagnosed as permanent who received no medical treatment. Ten percent of the youngsters who go through a screening program and have a hearing loss are found to have a permanent loss. This is what happens to the youngster who does not go to see his doctor when the hearing loss is discovered. We found out that 78 percent of them have either worse hearing or the same amount of loss. It is interesting that the numbers are almost identical—seventy-seven percent if they visit their doctor and 78 percent if they do not. So treatment as I have outlined it is important.

While giving this particular talk, which I have done several times, for example to the pediatric society here, I have had some interesting experiences. I am sure you people are familiar with these things. A screening test is done; if the youngster fails the test, a pure-tone audiogram is done. If he fails the pure-tone audiogram he goes to a school clinic where a physician—an otolaryngologist—checks the youngster, fills out a form, gives it to the parents and suggests that they go to see their doctor. If you see this form, treat it seriously. Or if you have to handle these forms, make sure that they are accurate. In my own experience, I have seen a youngster who came to me with a chronic otitis media, permanent perforation of the eardrum, and a very foul infection. In this instance, surgery was eventually required, not only to the nose and throat but also to the ear. At the first visit this child's father, who is a board-certified internist in the city of Detroit, reached into his pocket, pulled out this form, showed it to me and said, "Incidentally, I got this from school about ten months ago and I really didn't think it was important." And at that time, before the ear had started to drain and before there was a perforation in the eardrum, the child had a marked conductive hearing loss in that ear.

You all know this work is critical; continue to pay attention to it and treat it seriously at all times.

Chapter 5

SCHOOL SPEECH CORRECTION FOR CLEFT PALATE CHILDREN

MERVYN L. FALK

WE HAVE TALKED about the first three steps in an objective approach to cleft palate children; the term "objective" refers to the fact that with this being the means by which each person is working, there is no question as to where one might pick up somebody else's case should the original clinician have terminated with the case somewhere in progress. We also discussed the instructions as far as physiology and anatomy are concerned and the use of this normative body of information in relation to eliminating what is being done incorrectly to produce an abnormal speech signal.

We have mentioned, also, the role of sensory training, not only in terms of ear training, but insofar as visual, kinesthetic, and tactile training are concerned, as well as the relationship between the preliminary training and the eventual use of this training in the ensuing portion of the total therapy regimen.

We have also discussed the training of the organism, insofar as removing any physical causes are concerned, being carried out in tandem with the time devoted to the sensory training aspect of the program.

Note: Only the second of two lectures delivered by Doctor Falk is presented, since the substance of the first lecture is summarized in the second.

The total block of time spent on these three steps may be considered as a prespeech level of a total therapy regimen. Obviously, before you can train the child to utter something correctly, there has to be some background that he can use in order to do so. Otherwise, it puts you in a position, somewhat, as a parent who is very distraught by the fact the child substitutes /ɵ/ for an /s/, or blocks, or what have you, who says, "Johnny, don't do it this way, do it that way," and equates the child's ability to spontaneously correct his speech deviation with something such as sitting up at the table to eat or chewing food with the mouth closed. There has to be this preparation of the organism for the direct speech therapy portion of the total program. We consider this, then, to be a base from which to operate, a base from which the actual speech training level actually ensues; and as you are aware, there as yet has not necessarily been one attempt made by the child to produce a deficient sound correctly.

This begins with the fourth step and may well be the most important step of all that remains to be done. It is at this point that a person is taught to produce a sound correctly in isolation or with a neutral vowel. Just for the sake of clarification, I say with the neutral vowel in addition to the production in isolation, because we cannot produce all sounds in isolation. Some sounds, as you know, have to be produced with at least the neutral vowel.

If we think about the makeup of a heterogenous group and envision in this group six or eight children (as this somewhat typifies the size of your groups routinely) and put into this six or eight a cleft palate child, a stutterer, a voice problem, and a few different misarticulation types, then we might well have a rather realistic type of group before us. We are all aware that each of your groups will not have a cleft palate; each of your groups will not have a stutterer and each of your groups will not have a voice case.

We all know, too, that the vast, vast majority of the cases that need our help have so-called nonorganic misarticulation problems. I do not think we should necessarily take a view that these problems are nonorganic. I would hesitate to say that there isn't some organic basis for almost every speech problem; that is, organic or emotional. There has to be a reason why the child doesn't learn appropriately. We won't get into this much, but this is as opposed to the term "functional speech problem," which I think truly is a misnomer, particularly because the psychologists tend to have taken the market on the meaning of the term "functional." Certainly, all misarticulation problems with no organic base do not have a psychological or emotional base, either. So if we can distinguish between those that have organic bases and those that have nonorganic bases insofar as we know, then we are probably talking about the same animal.

Let me parenthetically state that I have thrown in the cleft palate child simply to meet the real tenor of why we are all here. There does not have to be a cleft palate child here, and the kinds of things that we will say will pertain to the cleft palate child just as they will pertain to the stutterer and just as they will pertain to the hoarse voice case. But we can think in terms of the cleft palate child as being present in this group because we will essentially be interested in working on this child's voice and articulation. We have tried to put this thing into a proper focus by indicating that there are really only three kinds of speech problems that you face in the typical school correction situation; these are of voice, rhythm, and articulation.

If for a stutterer we isolate particular sounds upon which he stutters, and we isolate for a cleft palate child sounds that he nasalizes, and if we isolate for the hoarse voice case sounds that he can produce without hoarseness as a point of departure for producing other sounds without hoarseness, and assign to each of the misarticulation cases specific sounds which they misarticulate, then we start to produce what is really a homogeneous group within this heterogeneous frame of reference. Keep in mind that we have defined the production of a speech signal as a modified voiced or voiceless airstream. Now what is done to overmodify or mismodify, as you might conceive of it, has really only to do with getting that child into the therapy situation.

From here on, we are interested in what is correct. Why do I say this? Well, think for a moment about the variety of misarticulated /s/ problems that you have. You talk about lateral lispers, you talk about interdental lispers, you talk about distorted /s/, you talk about nasalized /s/, etc. Yet, all you are teaching is a correct /s/; you do not really care if that child with a lateral emission for /s/ laterally emits the airstream, or if the child interdentalizes in order to produce an /s/, or if he allows that airstream for the /s/ to go through his nose; you're still interested in the so-called alveolar /s/. And all you are really interested in creating for the child, no matter what he does when he comes to you, is a correct articulatory position for him to assume each and every time he wants to produce the /s/ sound. And this is all we are talking about insofar as any speech problem is concerned.

Therefore, it doesn't truly matter whether the stutterer says "ba-ba-ba", or the lisper says "thither", or the cleft palate child says "s̃oap". We are still going to try and modify that voiced or voiceless airstream in such a fashion that the correct sound is produced insofar as our standards are concerned. This will be true, then, no matter what the nature of the diagnosis is; it does not matter if this child has a very gravelly, hoarse, harsh, breathy voice, or if he is overmodifying, or if he is substituting a /w/ for an /l/, or a /ə/ for an /s/, or an /&/ for an /s/, or whatever. All we are saying is that it doesn't matter what this child comes to you with; you are interested in normalcy. This is the whole substance of what we do. We teach a position within relative limitations for the correct production of a given sound.

We are saying, then, that if you put speech therapy in a heterogenous group on a rather pragmatic level, that each child in the group, regardless of his problem, will be dealt with in a fashion which permits him to receive as much therapy per day as each of the other members in the group.

It would appear that teaching correct modifications accomplishes this.

Subsequent steps in the speech training aspects of this total approach serve to reinforce and eventually to make automatic correct production of the sound first taught in isolation. Let us take a look, then, at the makeup of the group that we have structured for ourselves. We have a cleft palate child, a stutterer, a voice case, and assorted articulation errors. The sounds that you will be working with in the three misarticulation cases become obvious. With the cleft palate child, you will most often be working with one of the sibilant sounds or less often, plosive sounds. You will have to pick out, then, those sounds you are going to focus on for this child and it will always be in terms of what the sound is in automatic speech that he does not produce correctly. There may be a number of sounds that this child does not produce correctly in connected speech, but that he can produce correctly when you isolate a sound for him. We used the /s/ sound the other day as an excellent example where this so often happens.

One of the presuppositions here is that this child is in a state of readiness for speech correction class. The mere criterion of age, whether it be developmental or chronologic is not the only criterion. It should be rather obvious that the criterion is whether this child can achieve velopharyngeal closure or not. And what we so often find is that when the child is able to, that is, when the anatomy is sufficient, the physiology is not there. This child has apparently simply carried through into a period of his life following the surgical correction of this problem those patterns that he was using prior to surgical correction. Of course, surgery does not change neuromuscular patterns; all it does is move the anatomy around. So this child who, before pharyngeal flap surgery was saying s̃oap, might still say s̃oap, though when you isolate the /s/ sound for him and have him produce it in isolation, he might well produce /s/ quite normally. So this is the segment of

the cleft palate population that we're truly talking about—
that group that belongs in the speech correction class.

We mentioned that if the palate is short and the child
needs a flap, he really should not be in class; he should
be in the hospital getting a flap. And this is so true; you
are truly up against a brick wall when the child is unable
anatomically to achieve closure. For this moment you are
secondary; it is the child who is the one who is truly going
to pay, esssentially through the emotional route, for this
inability. We are talking about a child who belongs in your
room who is, then, essentially misarticulating. He has the
anatomy, the function is there, but you have to get it out.
What you do then is coordinate the elevation of the soft
palate with the coordinations that are necessary, essentially
of the tongue and mandible, so that when /s/ is produced,
the port is closed and the airstream is directed orally in its
entirety. What you end up with is a misarticulation case.
Keep in mind that the soft palate is an articulator; that in
the case where it anatomically is sufficient, you are dealing
with a misarticulation case.

This is not to say that during the "removal of physical
causes" phase you would not be using velar excercises, which
are the puffed-cheek drill, the gargling, the gagging, and so
forth, that we talked about. This is the prime place in which
to use these things. This is removing physical causes. Here
is a period of time that is devoted to this child strengthening
the musculature that has to be strengthened, so that when
he does go into the /s/ position, the palate elevates and
closure is effected. This is not to say, either, that you en-
capsulate each of these phases. This child with whom you
do these velar exercises, for example, may well continue to
do this many weeks beyond the point which you reach in
the teaching of a sound in isolation. But this involves a
home training program. You do not see him enough. You
recall this is something that has to be ongoing, day in and
day out, seven days a week, for from six months to a year.
You obviously are not the person to supervise this; the parent

is. And so you discipline the parent to how this should be done and then you put the child in his parents' hands.

At the same time, if the parent does not follow through, you have no recourse; you have to recommend flap surgery. For the case where the tissue is there and physiology is deficient, you use these exercises. This, also, will sometimes follow flap surgery for the child who still has air escaping because you have to strengthen the same musculature that comes in around the flap that you are strengthening in the case where there is no need for a flap but physiology is not yet intact. You are using the same exercises under the same condition of a rigid home training program, and meantime, you, back in the classroom, are dealing with the articulation phase of the problem.

If these children comprise the group, then, we assign the misarticulated sound in isolation to the part of the group that is essentially considered misarticulation; we assign a sound to the child with cleft palate repair—one which he is capable of producing in isolation if this exists; we assign to the stutterer a sound that he stutters upon; we assign to the voice case the /h/ sound. It is the only sound we assign him in isolation. We use the /h/ sound, first of all, because it has phonemic meaning. It is a phoneme; it is purposeful. We assign it, in addition, because it is produced through a relatively open glottis, and when the glottis is relatively open, it is in a relatively relaxed state. We use this as the sound in isolation because we are going to move to phonation from that sound when we get to combinations of sounds, and before we can expect this person to elevate his pitch, as is so often necessary with hoarseness, and produce through a relatively relaxed glottis in order to produce normal voice, we have to get this mechanism into a relatively relaxed state. And so we do it with the /h/ sound.

If, for example, we assign the /b/ sound to the stutterer, and in addition, we are dealing with /s,r,l/, we now have six sounds going for us. Let me say a word further about the stutterer to whom we have assigned a sound. Sensory training is important, physical causes must be removed, and it is necessary for the child to know physiology and anatomy. This is probably most true in the stuttering population. It is true with all of our cases; I do not mean to sell short the importance to any of them. But the stutterer has to be able to sense differences in lip pressure, tongue pressure, and these kinds of pressures of a physical nature of one structure against another. He also has to be aware of what it is he is trying to do, in general, from a physiologic standpoint. These backgrounds are particularly essential to the stuttering child.

There is not really a whole lot to say, then, at this point, beyond the statement of the rationale for assigning these children a sound with which to work. I would only offer that in the final analysis the speech signal is evaluated on the basis of articulation. You do not say a person has a speech problem because you evaluated his breathing, or you do not say that a person has a speech problem because you evaluated cerebration. You listen to him, and you listen to the *gestalt*, and the *gestalt* is not produced until this voiced or voiceless air stream is modified and emitted through one cavity or the other. Because both professionals and laymen do tend to base their judgments on the articulation aspect, it seems to become most critical to these people to focus on the modification portion.

You have dealt with respiration, you have dealt with phonation, you have dealt with resonation and cerebration in the prior stages; now you are ready to get into the articulatory stage, which leads, very simply, to the point that you can not fractionate this organism. You can not think just in terms of articulation therapy. If you are doing nothing other than filling a child in on some sound discrimination, you are training cerebration. If you are doing nothing more than coordinating respiration with phonation, you are working on respiration *and* phonation. Articulation, as the focus at this point, does not indicate that articulation is all that we are interested in. We are concerned with the total organism. We have held articulation until the rest of the organism is brought into the picture. Now we are going to superimpose articulation on the rest of the process, and we are going to bring five submechanisms together at this point and deal with the total system's production of a given speech signal.

We then move through subsequent steps which serve to reinforce and eventually make automatic correct production of the sound first taught in isolation. The fifth step, then, places the individual sound in combinations; that is, a sound is placed with a vowel in order to create a nonsense context so that no previously learned neuromuscular patterns are elicited. Typically, placing the consonant in the initial position then the final position and finally the medial position is advocated because in a simple to complex progression, this protocol is most consistent. When you have a person produce a particular sound in isolation, you are giving him as simple a context as you can. When he begins with that production and ends with a vowel, this is a bit more complex. Putting the sound being learned after a vowel would be the next. Finally, putting the vowel on each side of the sound being trained would be the most complex. Usually, we do it in this fashion rather than just taking an initial, medial, final sequence.

With the voice case who has learned to produce the /h/ through a relatively open and relaxed glottis, we combine /h/ with /ɑ/ because the child's mouth is already in position, insofar as articulatory relationships are concerned, to produce /ɑ/. This presumes that the /h/ is produced in isolation through a relatively open oral cavity which, in turn, has some secondary influence on the nature of the tonicity of the supralaryngeal musculature, the extrinsic musculature of the larynx from the larynx to the mandible. We have them wide open for the emission of a puff of air and then have them move to a vibratory position from the same articulatory position of production with an attempt to elevate pitch so that whereas the person has been producing /h/, the attempt now is for him to produce /hɑ/.

The most obvious indicator of success, probably, is when the child cannot phonate at first, which is a rather unusual way of relating to success. But what this indicates to you is that this child is attempting to produce voice in a different fashion, and this, of course, is what you are looking for. Whereas the hoarse voice is typically produced with relatively low pitch and you are attempting to have voice produced with some elevation in pitch, you would expect to get this kind of failure at first.

This is what is taken into other contexts in succeeding levels of the total regimen. Where we have a person doing this kind of thing, we move on to the use of vocabulary words where we try to reinforce patterns in context where there are previously established neuromuscular patterns. This person with the voice problem might now begin to produce such content as "one, two, three" with the new phonatory pattern, while at the same time, the stutterer is attempting to produce "boy"; the cleft palate child is beginning to produce "soap"; and the other children are talking about "running" and whatever else you may have them talk about. This, then, is the move into the sixth aspect of the total program where the new patterns for production of these sounds previously misproduced are utilized in context. Now you have everybody utilizing all of his previously acquired skills at the level of producing purposeful language.

We said earlier that producing the correct sound in isolation was probably the most critical aspect, and I think that this is true. It is also true, however, that when you start to integrate the correct articulatory pattern into the language pattern of the child, you are at an extremely critical point in the total therapy program for him. Now this child has to change some concepts, and this is a language function. He has to be concerned with "soup" starting with an /s/, not a /ə/; and he has to think in terms of "run" starting with an /r/ not a /w/, and so on. We are really talking about a language function at this point, in addition to the neuromuscular portion or the motor portion that we have been focused on to date. So again, proceeding from the simple to the complex, we would drill a number of specific words with the sound first in the initial position of a purposeful word, and then in the final position of a purposeful word, and then in the medial position of a purposeful word. Obviously, this would not be true in the voice case as much in the others because, for example, a final /h/ in a word is essentially not produced. We are, on the other hand, using other words with this person which would be compatible with his present level of ability so that it remains an ongoing, learning kind of experience; a situation, then, in which he is continually adding to his skills to produce voice through this relatively relaxed glottis.

The final step, which we have simply labeled "automaticity", is rather obviously the point at which we utilize such things as oral reading, conversation, the structured play situation, the structured social situation, and whatever we may think of as manifesting itself in the production of speech containing more than one word. This is something of which one particular point should be made. Too often, it would seem, we tend to dismiss the child before we have completed this particular aspect of the program. This might, for example, account for any of the regressions that we find children manifesting. Of course the real proof of the importance of this is the summer vacation, where you put so many on tentative or final dismissal at the end of the spring semester. However, when they come back in the fall, there is some semblance of the problem that they had before you dismissed them. This is probably the major indicator of the fact that we sometimes dismiss too soon. I think it is necessary that we spend as much time, or more, just at the level of automaticity as we do in the rest of the total program. When it takes you six months to get a child to the point where you can feel confident in having him attempt to integrate this new sound into connected speech, you might spend another six months reinforcing the use of that sound in connected speech.

The context which you use truly does not seem to matter

so much. It is much more important to get this child into a contextual environment with the sounds you have been working on; that is, in comparison with whatever the context itself may be. So to reinforce, we utilize any of those situations which we feel should be particularly meaningful to the child if he has some rather isolate sort of condition under which he should be functioning in a structured situation. In general, the typical speech correction class activities and regular classroom activities, in addition to the social situations each child faces, are sufficient. Once in a while you have somebody who returns to an unusual environment or reacts once he leaves the speech room in a rather unusual way in comparison to the way others will react when they leave. But, certainly, most children will benefit from the structured speech situation.

In summary, we have presented a formalized therapy format which first initiates the organism to the tasks inherent in correct sound production and then utilizes this background for correction of a specific deviation. Such an approach permits a clinician to proceed in an organized fashion to correct problems of several types when the premise of grouping is that it be by developmental age. This scheme allows the clinician to deal with articulation, rhythm, and voice, unencumbered by a need for real sophistication in psychotherapy or time to work very much on an individual level with cases whose basic problems are described in terms other than misarticulation.

Chapter 6

PSYCHIATRIC CONSIDERATIONS OF THE CLEFT PALATE CHILD

JOSEPH FISCHOFF

I WOULD LIKE to divide this up into more than one section. Not that it is separate, but I would like to talk about children first and then about the parents. But I am sure you all understand that as far as the child and the parents go, with children who are handicapped, they are pretty much one unit. The mother and the child especially, sometimes the father, are extremely important. But I think it is easier in terms of what is important in children to talk about them on their own. And I would like to talk at first in a very general way, because we have enough time to get into very specific things later, about children who are ill and children who have chronic handicaps over a long period of time and may have to live with them for the rest of their lives.

One thing that is very important is that a child does not separate the effects of the therapy from the effects of the illness. The by-products of the illness for any child are pretty much the same as the illness itself. The discomfort and the anxiety, the pain, the surgery, the shots, anything that a child gets at a very young age is very much the same as the illness, and so a child will not be able to thank you for what you do. He pretty much hates you for what you do and becomes rather passive and adoring if you are the doctor or a therapist because he is afraid of you. And this great admiration is pretty much an identification with the aggressor. But he better behave or he will be injured even more. And the more he does what you want, the sooner he gets out of your clutches. It is not a particularly adoring situation. The other extreme in early childhood, obviously, is where a child becomes extremely negative, very difficult to handle, and has to fight you tooth and nail in order to survive. He feels that he has very little autonomy and very little mastery over his body. He must fight to survive and keep whatever little bit of activity he has on his own.

Years ago, when we used to get children with polio who were in respirators, they would stop eating for the first two or three weeks. And it turned out to be that this was the only autonomous function that they had. They could open and close their mouth and refuse food or take it in. They had no control over every other bodily function, whether it was breathing, bowel movements, urinating, or even sometimes perspiration, depending on what was affected. After he stopped eating, the child would gradually begin to understand, sometimes with the help of the kid next to him who was in a respirator who had gone through it, what he was doing and why he was fighting back. Sometimes the fighting back can be self-destructive, but that would be very hard for a child to know. So, you can have two extremes in a child. One can be extreme passivity and subjecting himself to your every whim, and the other can be extreme aggression to obtain independence.

This is due to the child's own need to survive and the other has to do, of course, with what's going on inside of him. He can not really separate the feelings of illness and suffering from the action taken to cure him. And he can not comprehend really what is going on, as often adults can not really comprehend. Obviously, when a child is ill and has a congenital deformity, as with the cleft lip or cleft palate, the whole situation is different right from the beginning. And for a child, he at first is subjected to tremendous physiologic stress. Any child that has a congenital handicap to some degree is subjected to stress and tension beyond what is expected of an average newborn child in the first year or two. The tension often can be constant because it can have to do with difficulties in respiration, difficulties in eating, difficulties in swallowing, and a great deal of vomiting. We speculate that with the majority of infants, that any change early from a sleeping-eating pattern with intermittent wakefulness is discomfort.

Children with handicaps that they are born with have discomfort all of the time. This can often lead to a chronic kind of anxiety that is really without any later symbolic representation in the mind. It is a feeling of tension in the body that the person can not really ever put into words. You often see this, classically, when children have asthma where they can not ever say anything about what is wrong except that they are afraid they are going to die, they are afraid to be alone, especially without medicine. And one of the problems is that if it is not bound up tremendously in a psychological problem secondarily, this anxiety and this tension is *real* because the child with a congenital difficulty has it. You can not tell him that he is afraid of something that might happen to him in the future because it is something that has happened to him already. It is like telling a child whose mother has died that he does not have to be afraid that his mother is going to leave him; many kids are afraid their mother will abandon them and fantasize for the real reason. It is also like telling someone who has been in a terrible accident that he is really afraid of something that only happens once in a while. If it happens to you, it is very difficult for you to believe it is not going to happen again. So children who have extreme discomfort early, and there is not much in the way of a psyche very early—it is mostly a physiological reaction—eventually react to changes very rapidly and with great fear, especially. Of course we get into this later if the mother has reacted with the same kind of tension and anxiety early in the child's infancy.

The prolonged period of tension, defect, and anxiety also means that a child who has a handicap often has an extremely long period of dependency beyond what most children have. A great deal of this is normal; some of this goes into the area of being abnormal. But the handicapped child must turn to his mother and lean on her for many things in terms of the world that another child would not do. And this is something that can be very irritating to a mother or very gratifying because if she wants to keep the child close to her, this is one of the best ways to do it. The important thing to try to assess is how much of it is normal and how much is abnormal because this is where we get into many difficulties, since we initially asked the mother about the history and she will give certain things that sound like facts, but we are never sure whether these are or not. Often you have to assess this information by observing the child both in the office and in the home to understand what is really going on.

Another thing that happens to all children who have some type of handicap is that their body image is defective, though some studies say that this is not so. To skip ahead, one of the studies on children with cleft lip and palate shows that they drew pictures of the face that were just like other children, so body image was not defective. Well, that is a defective study because you get anybody with a severe type of handicap and when they dream about themselves they always dream about themselves as normal. They never have a defect in their dreams. You will never see a child beyond a very early age—of course they can not draw too well until they are at least four or five—who will ever draw a defect in themselves. They will draw a defect in anybody else but they will not in themselves. This kind of study is so naive, but I mention it because you are sure to read about it or maybe you have read it already. This has no validity at all. You cannot get children to draw themselves with defects if they have had them for a long time. If they have had it very quickly and suddenly, it is very traumatic. They will often draw themselves with a cast or with a bandage on their head. This is a very sudden onset of severe traumatic injury. A child with a long-term chronic defect will not draw himself as being abnormal. After all, he is fighting constantly to deny this and to be like everybody else. If you begin to treat him over a long period of time—and have many, many drawings over a long therapeutic relationship—eventually the child might draw himself as defective and still he might not.

But one drawing at one time about how a child looks is of no value at all.

As I said, all people who have handicaps dream of themselves as normal. And, of course, all children have basic wishes just to be very much like another child—like all the children. It is very frightening to a child to be very different than any other child unless he chooses to be so. In other words, he feels that he is as capable as all the other children. This need for competition and mastery becomes enormous. But sameness is very important to a child. And the sameness in his playmates and in his home, the repetition of very ordinary things, makes it very secure. If the child feels that things he has some control over do not repeat themselves and this happens often with a chronic handicap, it is very frightening because he does not know if the situation is going to turn out the same each time. And, obviously, in the early infancy of a child with a cleft, this anxiety about eating and breathing continues over a period of time also with the mother, and then the question of beginning to communicate becomes a major issue as the child gets older.

In a child's own life, he has many questions about why he has a defect. Things are not accidental in his life, so he has to have a reason for it. And as soon as he can begin to imagine, he might very well think that he was bad for one reason or another. Children who have had tuberculosis, diabetes, rheumatic fever, or orthopedic difficulties frequently have thought that they had this happen to them when, for some reason, they were bad. They do not know why, but the disease since time immemorial has been thought to be an affliction for being bad or transgressing in some way. The child will feel that besides his punishment, his mother may not love him as much because he is not perfect as all the other children. On the other hand, he may very well blame his mother for what is wrong with him. All children, early, blame their mothers for their sickness of any kind, whether it's an infected ear, a stubbed toe, or falling down and scratching the knee. It does not matter, because a young child who becomes hurt or injured, even if the injury is minor, can not take care of it himself. And if he can not, someone else has to take care of it immediately because he is in danger, since he does not know what he can do about this injury. The only person there is around most of the time is a mother or a caretaker and she must do it—she has to do it—in his own mind. This is his reasoning because he is so helpless and he is in danger and she can stop it. So, if she does not stop it she is to blame. We frequently see children who have an acute illness and before they can even begin to verbalize, they will hit their mother. If they have, for instance, an acute, severe diarrhea and the mother goes to pick them up, they will strike out at her—they will strike out at anybody—partly because they feel she is in a conspiracy to make him feel so bad. I have frequently seen a child who was around three and had his tonsils out tell his mother that he hated her, go away, and she is to blame for what happened. And not that this was something not understood because many of them had the situation explained to them—they understood it—and they shook their heads. Children understand very little, by the way, and you should never be deceived by what they say they understand. What they tell you in words has very little meaning. They parrot it back to you because they know that is what you want them to say. And as long as they say it, you will like it and you will be pleased. And it is very important that they please you and so you believe they really understand. A mother will explain to her child that he is going to have his tonsils out, and he goes, and then he becomes infuriated at her because his throat hurts so much. And he tells her to go away and never come back and he hates her. Of course the pain goes away in the next day or two, but during that time it is pretty severe. So, a child always blames the mother for the illness. He has to because there is nobody else to blame. But in addition he is terrified at the loss of the support and the care that he needs that only a mother can give. So, he has to weigh that, also. Thus, the normally ambivalent relationship that any child has toward a parent, and any parent has toward a child, is obviously much more stressful in a child with a congenital handicap or an illness that may occur later.

We always talk, of course, about ambivalent relationships that children have toward their parents. I think that's primarily because the children can not talk about the ambivalent relationship the parents have toward a child. They do not write the books, and they do not make the speeches. Every parent has mixed feelings about their child and every child has mixed feelings about the parents. It is very acceptable to write in books that children love and hate their parents and everybody now accepts that as common knowledge until his own child does it to him and then it is very special knowledge and it is very different than the book. But the ambivalent relationship that a parent has toward a child is very important, especially, in a child with a long-term handicap. I remember a mother who had a child with severe cerebral palsy and would faint very often in the middle of a street, and she had recurrent dreams of this boy. He was multiplied many times over and in the dream, all of these images of him were always dead. And this is what she wished—that he were dead. And her fainting had very much to do with wanting to be taken care of herself because he required enormous amounts of care. But she always had to smile and say it never bothered her, while actually she hated it and she wished she had not had him, which would be a normal acceptance of any situation like this. But since she was always supposed to be a good mother, this was unacceptable so that this is how she would solve her problem—by fainting and dreaming. She often said she could not understand why she always dreamed about him dead. It might surprise you, but parents always, or often, will not want to be aware of what it is. Did he die? Was it accidental? Did someone kill him? But you have to point out to parents that nobody created this dream but themselves so that perhaps they did want him dead.

That was not an unusual situation, and children with severe handicaps are so different to their mothers when they first have them—they have to be. In reality, as opposed to fantasy, no mother imagines she is going to give birth to a defective child.

However, a very common dream toward the end of pregnancy is one in which the mother dreams of death, but that really is not death. It has to do with separation of a part of her that is going to leave her—the newborn baby. But many mothers are afraid of that dream because they think they want the baby to die or they are going to die. But since death has nothing to do with our imagination, since none of us know what it is to die but all of us know what it is to be separated, often dreams that have to do with death have to do with separation. So, those are not quite the same.

On one hand, children will blame the mother for their defect and on the other hand they are afraid that the mother will get rid of them and not like them as much. Thus they are often caught in a bind and frequently they become the good child. This is the pseudo-adult child who does things in terms of ego development quicker than other children, because in this way they show their mother that they are worth something and in this way they also feel that they, themselves, are more capable and that they can please their mother. It is a more overt form of a case in which children show off because the parents want them to show off.

Other things happen, too, in a child who has a congenital handicap. There is repeated attention and manipulation, surgical and otherwise, to one area, so that often this one area becomes exceedingly important—beyond what it would in normal development. Technically, you would say that this area is hyperdefective, that everything centers around the mouth and the palate and the functions of swallowing and breathing and communication. With a child with a clubfoot, everything centers around the foot, and every change in that area becomes a major issue. The whole world is focused in this one area. This is natural because any of you who have had a filling fall out of a tooth, leaving a hole, put your tongue there and it is the whole world. You have a little bit of pain there and everything else is unimportant—the whole of your life centers around this one temporary illness until it is fixed. You do not care about anything until the temporary pain and discomfort go away. You have a minor rash on your skin and the world sort of dissolves, especially if there is a minor discomfort associated with it, until that rash is taken care of. Well, imagine a child who has constant chronic discomfort and he lives with this. He does in many ways. As I say, everything centers around it, whether he knows it or not.

Another thing that he learns because he has had this chronic pain, discomfort, and physical deformity for a long time is to live with that level of pain that would be almost intolerable to a normal child—I mean physically normal; I don't mean psychologically. You see this with adults who have chronic pain such as severe back pain, severe pain from chronic illnesses that are internal. You would never know they have the pain because they have learned to live with it. They have not adjusted to it; they are living with the pain and the pain is always there and the discomfort is there. You ask them how they feel and they say fine. And what are they going to do? Sit you down and tell how much they hurt? And you do not really care because there is nothing you can do about it, either. You can care about it in the sense that you feel bad that they have it, but there is nothing you can do about it, either. So many children very quickly learn this—and they live with that level. But do not fool yourselves that they are not constantly adjusting to a certain degree of stress that is more than other children have to adjust to. It often can promote great changes in terms of mastery of the environment and ego development later on because they have learned that you have to live with certain things and do as much as you can to alter the situation. Thus many children with a handicap do extremely well later on in terms of handling the world and adapting to it because they have had to adapt to other extremely adverse circumstances. You see this with kids with hemophilia, for instance. Everytime they bump a door they get a tremendous bruise on their elbow, or they cough hard and something ruptures in a joint and they bleed. They learn to live with this over a long period of time, but they feel like they are sitting on a time bomb and they are! These children become extremely sensitive and acute to the world around them because they have become that sensitive to themselves. Frequently they can become very sensitive in certain fields and be able to work very well, because they are alert to changes and really externalize what they have learned from long experience internally so that they make great use of this in terms of their vocation later on.

But the whole area of the body does become the most important part for a long, long time, and it must be that way until finally a child learns that he only has to pay attention to it in times of stress or when he senses that it is way beyond what should be normal. It takes a long time for the child to understand how far his body has to go out of commission before it is normal or abnormal. Early in life, it is immediate. As soon as his body is not doing well, he is terrified and immediately is upset and goes to his mother. On the other hand, a child who is older and can communicate more can tolerate more and more stress. You know, inhibitions in certain parts of the body can cause you much difficulty. For instance, children who are immobilized for a long period of time often develop tics in their face, blink their eyes, twitch their nose, curl their hair, or scratch other parts of the body because there has to be motor discharge if verbal communication is still limited. In the very young child, there are other movements and you should not be concerned about them, so that with a child who has a cleft you may get many other movements early; you may get much more motor activity, and because verbal communication is limited and he can be quite active for a long period of time, it is nothing to be concerned about.

In addition to the defenses against being very passive— and this is where clinical assessment is important—what is normal and what is not normal? I think these are important issues. Usually, the activities you see in early childhood are all overdetermined. There is not a one-to-one relationship, even early. And so, to attribute one cause to one activity all the time is not correct. It is usually an overdetermined activity, so that you may have five or six reasons why a child is doing something. The important thing is to pick out the one that is important at the time. Is it the mother? Is it the child himself? Is he active because he is rebelling against her? Is he active because he is brain damaged? Is he active because he has some fantasies at night? There are many reasons for why. Is he in great pain? And is he doing this for that reason? But it is somewhat naive always to pick out one cause for one action except that in certain ages, in certain levels of development, you expect a child to act a certain way. So, it might be more important at one age. For instance, eighteen months to two years is an age of great negativism and opposition, so that when you ask a child if he wants a cookie, he says, "No!" And then he looks, he thinks about it, he says, "Yes!" And then he takes it. But it is an age where he has to take and he can not be given to. So at that age, if you get more opposition, you know that you usually expect it and it probably has very little to do with the mother or anything unusual. But if you get it at four and five, and you get it as a constant characterologic way of life, there is something wrong.

There are usually several reasons for why a child is acting a certain way. The significant thing is to pick out the one that we think is important right then. And that sometimes requires a great deal of talking with the mother or the father. Certain kinds of procedures are experienced in different ways. I know early surgery is not experienced as anything in the mental life of a child, but certainly from nine or ten months on, it is experienced as a great catastrophe and a kind of mutilation and total annihilation. This is how children think—it is either all or none—so when they wish you were dead or say it, they do wish you were dead, but you are going to come back anyway. So, it does not matter and children really do not see the inevitability and permanence of death until they are about nine years old, so they can kill you off many times and you still are all right. Children can experience major irreversible catastrophes in their own fantasy many times, too, and in reality, this is the end of the world. You should understand that certain events do have an effect on them. There are catastrophic events in childhood and they do have a great deal of effect on the child. Later on, the total catastrophe is more and more circumscribed to having something done to them because they deserve punishment and they were bad. And as they develop more of a conscience around three, and as they get a little older—four and five—then it often has to do with castration anxiety; that there is retaliation for whatever they imagine they are going to do to their own father. But, you see, there is a gradual circumscribing of the areas that are going to be hurt. An example is the child who had been operated several times on his penis for hypospadias and other malformation, and by the time he was five he was determined that he was going to be a penis doctor. And you know what he is going to spend his life doing in his fantasy is probably cutting them all off because in his own imagination this is what was always happening to him. This is what I mean. He can have this major catastrophe over and over and over again. It does not matter to him that he comes out whole each time. In his imagination, before the surgery, it is going to happen again. In surgery, five times before five is a lot. So he was sure he would be a urologist but did not know the word for it.

Among other reactions that children have, I would emphasize the defense mechanisms. Obviously, all of these defense mechanisms are normal because they exist in everybody's life all of the time. The degree that these exist in a child is what is important. You often see an increase, for example, in denial, where in the study to draw a picture they didn't draw the picture of an abnormal face. There always has to be an increase in the denial in any child that has a congenital abnormality. Children deny most of the world, normally, when they are young, anyway. They feel that what is no good does not exist or it is not in them and it does not belong. Denial is a normal way of life for children. Therefore, the important thing is how much more denial exists. And as life goes on, it is important to deny certain areas that are not capable of change, anyway. You work with the areas that are good. So denial is one mechanism that is increased.

Another defense mechanism is isolation. The whole area is just put away and circumscribed and does not exist. I have mentioned identification with the aggressor and the aggressor is the mother. It can be the doctor, but it has to be the mother, too. She is the all-powerful witch who is causing all the trouble in addition to all the good that she is doing. And I am sure you have all seen the regression—that the child must go backward under stress, and again, this is a normal type of defense mechanism. Often, at the critical stages of development, children at certain developmental stages, at eighteen months, two and a half years, sometimes three and a half will often have a regressive period. It is temporary, and it disappears. The child might go back to baby talk, or wetting, or other infantile behavior, sometimes with the developmental stage from the internal development. Sometimes it is due to a move or to an illness at home, or some catastrophe, and they may regress temporarily.

The other defense mechanism has to do with the reaction formation—denying anything that has to do with the illness and developing a Pollyanna attitude toward life. Everything is wonderful; nothing is wrong; I just do not know what you are talking about when you say that I may have trouble about this, or would worry—just completely avoiding the problem. Denial can work in some important ways because often the denial is not just the denial that the child has to do. The mother sometimes will minimize the child's congenital handicap to such a degree that the child, when he looks in the mirror, has real trouble in believing his own eyes. And the mother keeps saying that it is not that bad, it is unimportant, and that he shouldn't worry about it till there is such a discrepancy in his perception of what is real that the child gets confused about reality. What I am saying is that there has to be a very realistic explanation to parents that this is what exists and this is what is seen and this is what the child is going to see, also. The mother wants to protect the child and wants to minimize it and will say about a child who speaks very, very poorly and cannot be understood by other children on the block, "Well, you can understand him—I can." Well, she can. She also communicates with him on a nonverbal level and, besides, has lived with him a long time, but if others cannot understand him, they cannot. Often they can. But it is this kind of thing—he is like everybody else and there is nothing different about him—which can distort a child's sense of reality to the point where he cannot really believe his own ability to figure out what is going on.

So, there is always an increase in fantasy life in children who have defects. They are often fantasies that have to do with being very athletic—perfect, you know, heroic and great—especially in those children who are handicapped to the degree that they are just immobilized. They become, in their fantasies, the greatest of all, so it is very important not to feel that children are going out of the bounds of normal when they imagine these things. They want to. If you let them talk about it, they eventually will tell you. They know it is not real and it is not possible, but they wish it were. Also, there is always the wish for magic—that sometime in the future there will be some medical method discovered that will do away with whatever medical handicap they have. I think you always have to be very honest in saying this is all that can be done at this time and nobody knows if something more will happen later on. You know, if you say maybe and perhaps, this is terrible, because you do not know. If you really do not know, you say that at this time this is what can be done. Many people are afraid to say this because they are afraid of inflicting pain or sorrow or causing somebody to be sad. But if you leave somebody with a false hope, you do them a great deal more harm. They do not accept what they have got and will often be very depressed and hoping, "Why didn't it come now" and, "I should be better." You have to help them adjust to what is realistic today. If something does happen that is better, that's great. But you can also cause them to go on a rat race all over the country, seeking help where there isn't any help and cause untold harm both financially and emotionally to many families by offering hope that is nonexistent. It is very rare that one place, when a handicap is very common, has the answer over all the other places. Sometimes it is true, but that is the exception— that isn't the reality. You have to say that this is as much as can be done at the present time and if you are conversant with the field, you are usually right that nothing great has happened in the last twenty-four hours that you would not know. Once in a lifetime you may be wrong, but I don't think you should always leave the door open; this magical feeling exists in everybody who is ill. Patients with cancer know they are going to die and that is all there is to it. Everybody wants to feel that a handicap is going to be reversed completely. I think this is what people live in the hopes of.

The social aspects of the child with a handicap are extremely important. Generally I believe that children that are handicapped should be put in a social situation very early. I think preschool nurseries are great. If there are lots of children on the block and there is a lot of junk around in an empty lot and the children can play, they do not need to go to preschool nursery, but with the way land is being taken up, it is hard to find an empty lot, or an alley, or junk, except garbage. But, a socialization experience very early is important for a handicapped child. First, he learns that other people look at him and ask about him and he learns how to handle that. He has learned how to do it from his mother, but he expects his mother to be that way; she has to take it whether he is good or bad; she is not going to kick him out, and he finally believes that. But he does not really know how other people are going to accept him outside of the mother and the relatives. So he should be with other children early. It is also good for the others because they learn how to look at a child who is different and live with him and not be frightened. Out of all the questions that other children ask, some have to do with being different, but the basic issue has to do with, Will it happen to me? And that is terrifying for any child. After all, if it could happen to him, it can happen to me.

Thus a child has to get out with his mother into a group of children, early if it is possible, and into the community. But you do get the other side—that mothers tend frequently to overprotect children with a handicap. They do with orthopedic defects and they do with children with severe speech deficits and with clefts because they are afraid the child is going to be exposed to emotional injury, that people will laugh and the parent will frequently talk for the child. Someone has to question him; before the child can open his mouth, his mother has put all the words into it. And the mother says he cannot do something but often he can do more than she gives credit for. Sometimes they will go to the extreme of putting on his clothes longer than they should. Eating is something that does not become independent for a long time. So I always ask questions about all different areas, not the one that is just related to the handicap, when I talk to parents about their child. What can he really do? You know, can he ride a tricycle, or is she afraid to let him try to ride a tricycle because he has some other difficulty in some other area? Or if he will fall down and get hurt. Is she afraid that she would feel more guilty if he gets injured in some other area that she just has to wrap him up and keep him like a little baby? Generally you will find that mothers of handicapped children do limit the number of experiences that they allow their children compared to the nonhandicapped. And this, of course, decreases the child's feeling of being independent and feeling capable. It works in a very vicious circle. And it is hard for a mother when she feels her child is suffering, and often she feels that he is suffering way beyond what he is, to watch him struggle to accomplish something that another kid can do very easily. But she has to let him struggle with it. You often hear normal children tell their mothers or fathers that they want to do something themselves. And their parents' excuse is, you know, it is going to turn out a mess and I am going to have to redo it. But how is a child going to learn to do anything unless you watch him? Although he is pounding a nail into a board and the nail gets all battered up and the board gets a mess and he finally gets the nail in but then you have to pull it out and put it in straight, he is very proud of what he did. It takes longer for a child with a handicap but it has to be done in exactly the same way. Children do not like to be done for, they like to make their own mistakes, because by making their own mistakes they feel they are very capable. So this is significant.

Another thing that has to do with social acceptance is that in one study, children were asked what boy or girl do you like best and they had six drawings. (This study has never been repeated. I think it would be interesting if it were.) The first was nonhandicapped and that was the child who was accepted by the others easiest on drawings or pictures; second, they accepted a child with a leg brace and crutches; third was a child in a wheel chair; fourth, a child who had a congenital amputation of the left hand; then the child with a slight facial disfigurement; and then the obese child—I guess nobody likes a fat kid. But I would like to see that study repeated. It is significant that people are at first quite in awe of anybody who has a facial disfigurement. Whether it is a cleft or scars on other parts of the face, they are very upsetting, very frightening, to them. Anything above the neck, to humans, is extremely important. This is the area that is more important than any other part of the body because it contains the brain. It also contains their identity—their face. At least you begin to feel very early that your face is you. This is not true, because many skilled observers can tell by somebody's walk or posture who it is—they may not even see them, yet they know who it is. But to a child—and this lasts all the rest of your life—it is the brain that is the most important and your face is you. Thus, any distortion in your face is terrifying. People resort to a very quick regression when they see a distortion in a person's face, because they immediately feel, again, that if it happens to them, it can happen to me. And this is a very frightening thing.

This is getting into the difficulties that children with clefts have. They look different and other children are afraid of this possibly happening to them. And why did it happen? Therefore, the social acceptance of the child is something that I would urge very, very early and without a doubt as being one of the most important areas of all. What has to do with facial disfigurement is much more important than what has to do with a clubfoot or a hand that is deformed. Internal things are unimportant to children because they cannot conceptualize them, but external deformities are very important even though they are often less life threatening than internal deformities. After all, you can rarely see any external manifestations of leukemia, but it does kill little children. You see only minor external manifestations when they are close to dying, but that is unimportant to people and unimportant to children. The face that is so important is the one thing that, of course, children with clefts show so clearly, and it is very upsetting to them. Even when a kid without a cleft gets braces on the teeth, just to straighten his teeth out, the first thing he is called in school is metal mouth or rabbit or robot, and that is what they are called immediately.

If you minimize the fear, it is very, very important. Many years ago I fractured my neck and had to be in a brace for a number of weeks. Every once in a while I would walk down the street and I guess that I should not have, but a child would look at me and cry and run away. It was obviously terrifying. I must have looked like a monster he had seen on television or in the movies. No questioning about what it was, or what was it for, or that I was walking down the street with two kids, one on each hand—that was unimportant. Obviously, those kids were surviving, but when they saw this horrible vision, they immediately would run away and cry—both boys and girls. The boys would try to be more brave, but it did not last very long, until they got used to you. I was not that different, but anything becomes enormously important to people and they turn away from it in revulsion because of their own fears of it happening to themselves. It is the people who can separate themselves from this and see it for what it is who then have no great fears of the situation and can handle it realistically. Obviously, if you deal with people in therapy, this is what you must do. You cannot always be the good one who is going to take care of them and sympathize with them and pat them and keep them infantile. They will never grow. This is what people do not understand very well when they are always asking questions and always want to be overprotective.

I have tried to make this whole discussion of handicap a rather general one, not because I have not worked with kids with clefts and with severe speech difficulties, but because you cannot pick it up purely as something unique if you have worked with children with all kinds of handicaps as I have for a number of years. The handicap is something in addition and something special when it is a cleft in a certain way. But what I am trying to emphasize is all the ramifications that are not special at all, and I would say there are close to 90 percent that are not special. Where you can take advantage of it being unique is where you can work with a whole group of parents who have children who have had the same difficulty. We work with parents whose children have all been burned and they have a common guilt and depression and anxiety to work out. We work with the mothers in groups where the children have all had epilepsy. Working with groups of mothers and fathers where the children have a common illness is not a bad idea. In fact it is a very effective one because on one level they all share the common fears and anxieties that other people just cannot share because they do not have anything like this. There are also practical problems when a child has a handicap that the parents can help each other with. This can apply to anything in terms of literature or where you buy something or how you handle the situation at home. There are the fantasy problems of the worries about what will happen to the child and how far you go, so that working with groups of parents becomes technically a very good kind of therapy. They support one another and often mothers have worked out practical, technical solutions that you really have not thought of, but they have been innovative and have worked it out very, very well. So, we often will group mothers according to disease, but that is not because of the mothers themselves. It is really because of the handicap that the child has; here the mothers do support themselves.

The immediate concern that mothers have when a child is defective, is that, as I mentioned earlier, they are very anxious and frightened. They are hurt, disappointed, helpless, and very resentful, and may be ashamed and feel very guilty. They wonder why the child was born this way, and no amount of intellectual explanation is really helpful, except you should give it because the mother has the need. Often these feelings are buried very early by feelings that become rather altruistic on the surface, such as compassion and love and taking care of the child. The mother really wants to make restitution in terms of feeling that something that she has done has created this child and also that she, herself, will be an adequate mother. She feels that if she gave birth to a child who is defective, there must be something wrong with her. So, as I said when we began, we just cannot talk about only the child, we just cannot talk about only the mother or the father—it is all one unit in the family and it does involve the other children, too.

There have been some studies at times about parental adjustment, how the mother is adjusted and whether they were better or worse; some studies have said that the mother seemed to undergo more stress and more maladjustment than the father. What happens frequently is that the child can serve as a scapegoat at the wrong time. You see this often with a mother who is wrong—and they become a scapegoat; they become the one who is handicapped emotionally. It is pretty much axiomatic that an environmental crisis, change, or stress often serves as a focus for family trouble to react to. They can all react to this now and say, "That's the trouble," and minimize the trouble that is really underneath. This is very common. And they all say, "Now if we could solve this environmental situation, we would not have any other problem at all." So, if you are trying to work with a mother that is overly concerned about certain details—the child's behavior, rearing the child, how she should handle your instructions that you are giving—you just wonder why she is asking so much. You can be fairly sure that it is not about the child, that there is something else that is plaguing her besides this, and there are other troubles at home besides her concern about how to manage her child who has a cleft.

Other studies have shown, but they are mostly Minnesota paper and pencil tests, that there is no difference between children who are normal and children who are chronically disabled in some other way than children who have this cleft lip. Another person said that there was no correlation between speech proficiency and adjustment, again on the basis of the Personality Adjustment Test. Because the things we are talking about are extremely involved, we can't always trust paper-and-pencil tests. I think that they are one means of evaluation, but they cannot really replace the interview that you must have because this is where you get most of what is going on underneath.

But the drawing is great. You draw a person—you draw a family, a house, a tree, and a person. They are all fine, but they won't really serve as a substitute for knowing the family and the history of the family and of the child. What many professional people do is make a technical error of imagining that the parents are going to be the sole therapist, that they are going to understand the situation and do what you say. They know what is going on. They shake their heads "yes" and go home and carry things out just right. But this is not true. The parents have a child with a handicap, it is a catastrophe for the parents, and they have to work through their own problems before they can begin to carry out your directions. They can carry them out in a very defensive fashion in terms of meticulous care, but they can be obsessive about it and then this is of no great value either because it displays their own anxiety.

I can list a number of things that parents are very concerned about very quickly with their children when they have a facial deformity such as cleft lip. They are concerned immediately about the appearance of the child; whether they admit it or not, that is the gravest concern of all. They are concerned, secondly, about the desirability because it can work both ways. They can want surgery immediately and feel, "Now we will get rid of it—no one will know about it, and we won't have any more trouble." On the other hand, they may see this as a great and grave injury and insult to the child because they are so vulnerable and they are afraid of surgery. So do not assume because they are asking about when surgery can be done, that they are saying to you, "We want it right now," or, "When will it happen?" They may be very terrified of what will happen to that child undergoing surgery. They are very concerned early about how the speech will be, and they are very frightened that the lip will not turn out well. They want reassurance that it will and you cannot give that immediately. You can give it in terms of experience—numbers; a child with this kind of difficulty; if it heals well; what it might be; but you cannot say immediately what it will be.

The parents are greatly concerned about feeding because they are frightened that the child will aspirate and die. Mothers are very concerned about their ability to feed a baby and they are very worried; and the mothers are always very worried about what the fathers are going to think, what the husband's reaction is going to be. It can be a very accepting one, but it can also be one of great rejection—perhaps of himself for his ability to be a father. He can blame his wife, that she caused it, you know, and it is from her side of the family, and she had the pregnancy, so it must be all her fault. He forgets that he had something to do with it; very convenient for a man. But, mothers are very concerned about how the father will accept it. And, then, the mothers are worried about how the other children will take it. As I said, children who are exposed to other children early who are handicapped take it very well. They have no problem, because they had the problem initially and they worked it out very quickly. And so they do accept it; they do not reject it. Then, of course, there is worry about friends and family and what will they think and what will they do? They also worry about the child's intelligence. Is something that shows on the outside a sign of a defect in the brain? Well, obviously, most of the time it is not, but sometimes it is, although this is not the common circumstance. It is unfortunately axiomatic that a child with one type of congenital anomaly often has another one. If a child has one anomaly, he has one somewhere else. He has a predisposition because usually anomalies occur at certain levels of development in the fetus, so that many systems can be vulnerable at the same time. But I will go into that more in terms of intelligence.

The financial aspects are important, too, and parents worry about it. They hide it from you and do not do anything, but they do worry, rightfully, because any kind of disability costs a lot of money. They do not know about state aid or other things that are available—most people do not. And they are worried about whether this defect or some other defect will occur in unborn children in the future. This is a realistic fear. You hear so much about genetics, and only someone who knows about genetic counseling would know that if there are other defects in this child how other children might be affected. But many parents are very frightened that their child will not be able to speak at all and to really communicate. So the parents need a great deal of counseling before there is any surgery.

Some time ago, we were asked to work with one clinic

in cleft palate and cleft lip with kids who were twelve and thirteen years old because they are adolescents or preadolescents and they are beginning to act up. And it took, surprisingly, quite a bit of conversation to point out that the counseling of these families should go back a long, long way. The people in charge of the clinics were interested and concerned about doing something about these kids at this time and really had said they had adjusted fairly well over a period of years and now they seem to be acting up and not accepting what they were and were disciplinary problems. We have to start early because this is where a great deal of prevention can be done. For instance, their concerns with the cleft lip and palate are greater than the parents with a child that has only a cleft palate, because the external deformity shows, and so the parents, even though it may be in the end less of a problem, are more concerned if the lip is involved. And the questions that the mother and father have are different. The father will emphasize less physical acceptance; competency becomes important to a man. To a mother, the appearance is very important. She does not want the child to be hurt. They both want the child to be accepted. And the mother feels that the child is very fragile and vulnerable. So the concerns of the parents are quite different. The father can minimize and deny the handicap; in fact, he may overemphasize the competence of the child and push him faster than he should. This is where parents start to get into trouble because they do not agree on what should be done.

Another study had to do with psychological adjustment of the parents of children who had cleft lips and palates and used a control group of normal children and normal parents in terms of physical normality, not emotional. I have found that the parents of children who have clefts are more anxious and concerned. I think their conclusions were these: the parents of older handicapped children seem to be even more anxious in terms of the younger children and concluded that the effects develop with time. But this is so difficult to really assess in that all parents of all adolescents have troubles.

I think that this is something you can't quite say so openly—
that as the child gets older the parents get worse. Just playing into the adolescent's hands, then, they will never learn,
but I think that in adolescence the child with a cleft, if it
is quite visible and there is a speech difficulty, does become
very upset.

This is why the clinic, as I talked about, is having trouble,
because they are getting a lot of adolescent children at a
period when social acceptability becomes very important.
This has been where mothers become very upset with their
daughter or son; he seems to be less acceptable. The mother
then begins to feel that she is doing a poorer job than she
really is. And she really may not be doing such a poor job.
This may be an internal struggle that the child has to go
through and finally come to terms with, but it is not necessarily true that the mother or father is not being an adequate
parent. During the turmoil of adolescence, the child's image
that he has constructed of himself in latency is pretty solid
and then normally is dissolved because he has to look at himself very differently as he changes physiologically. His whole
body is changing; there is a relative ego weakness in each
adolescent child compared to the upsurge of the drive. So
some parents may feel that they have been very competent
and have had a fairly adequate adjustment with their child
with a handicap in latency. But suddenly they feel that
they are utterly inept—that they have taken all of the responsibility for what is happening in adolescence where this
may not be the case at all. That this is more severe for a
child with a handicap is often true.

Diabetic children will often have to deny a defect and they
stop watching their diet and will come in in a coma. It is not
unusual for a child to go through this two or three times in the
middle adolescent years and finally become more introverted.
So, you see, certain defects are much more dangerous for life
than others. The girls will feel that with a defect like this, they
are unacceptable to anybody so they may as well die. The boys
will feel they are weak and therefore they will have to deny

that they are diabetic and will come in in a coma. You can thus see the need for denial of any kind of deficiency in adolescents, both in normal adolescents and those who have a handicap that is extreme. Here you have to consult the parents and find out that it is nothing that they are doing, particularly, that this is their child's way of behaving and that he has been very upset just recently.

Now I would like to say something about the intelligence of the cleft palate children and their parents and the examiner who does the different studies. First, I will discuss one study where children were retarded in varying degrees. On the WISC, the cleft palate children had a mean IQ of 94. The verbal skills were less, as you would expect; they were eleven points lower. Performance skills were about seven points lower. The researchers who administered the test said that in the natural distribution, you would expect 25 percent to have below 90 IQ. But, of the children with a cleft, there were 40 percent. One of the problems in this kind of study is that since a variation of ten points one way or the other on the WISC is meaningless, we then pinpoint things like eleven points or seven points, and in reality, there is no problem. And this is very important because any one child from year to year can get a ten-point variation. You would have to get a wide discrepancy, twenty points or so, at least, to really begin to say that these tests have some meaning. And this is where too much is placed on numbers. You could draw all kinds of conclusions that should not be drawn on the basis of those test scores. A conclusion of another study was that children with good rehabilitation services, when they were compared to their siblings, were only a few points different, which, of course, means no difference; and that their long-range achievement in language and social adaptation in school was good.

Another study, this one concerned with creativity, found differences in the sense that cleft palate children seemed to be less creative. This was attributed to overprotective, rejecting, or overstriving attitudes of the parents which may or may not be so, but there have not been many studies done like this. I think that creativity in children is very difficult to assess, especially in latency between seven and eleven. So, the creativity part was a very small part of the study and I do not think it took latency into account.

Another study that had to do with social competence found that as the children got older, in the families that were fairly well adjusted, they approached normal children in social competence but there were more pronounced difficulties in children below five and six than there were with older children. The children frequently have shy and retiring qualities till they get to know you; they do not have that shy, retiring quality with their friends on the block. This is why it is so often important to see what a child is like at home, with his playmates or in his nursery. They are self-conscious of their appearance and this you would expect. Perhaps there might be, in addition, an inability to function on tests and in school because of their feelings that they have to hold themselves back; and there is a worry and feeling that they are not competent. But very often I have seen this really pop when the parent's great concern is that their cleft children are not competent. You can quote all kinds of studies. One said that they were as competent as everybody else; another said that they were not. One study said that they were lower; another study said that they were not, that there was not that much rejection. And these are repeated things that have gone on since about 1946. Each is saying something different, but on clinical evidence you see the great concern the girls have about adolescence, and kissing and dating, and whether they will be acceptable in marriage. And they say it very, very openly.

It does not help to tell an adolescent girl that the majority of women who have had the same difficulty are married; that does not apply to her and it never does to any adolescent. It is also true that it does not do any good for a parent to tell an adolescent that they have been through it, too. Well, "that was in the olden days." And, "you don't understand." You have to understand the internal problem of the child, and the mother's great distress is that maybe her daughter won't be accepted; this is very, very frequent. The daughter senses it, too. Then you get into real battles over things that are unimportant, things that have nothing to do with the basic issue of the stress that is going on. It has to do with whether the daughter will be acceptable to everybody. As I said, the mother's concern has to do with aspirations of being acceptable. The father is concerned more with conquering the world. One author says that the professional and middle class with higher aspirations might be more disheartened over their child's not functoning as well, but I have never found this to be so. They may be more verbal and make more noise about it, but I think that the other groups in the lower class are just as concerned, frightened, and disheartened. They may be much more fearful because sometimes they cannot put their questions into the form that you can understand about the worries and the fantasies, and the exceptions or lack of exceptions, about the children. I have found that the children who will have the greatest difficulty in the adjustment have a reflection of disorganization of the family.

Early counseling is really a primary counseling, a kind of primary prevention. You do not wait for something to occur. If you could have it the way you would like, you would like it to begin right after the baby is born and identified. Sometimes this kind of help can take different forms. For instance, at first, counseling is rather intensive, where you will talk with the parents frequently over a period of months, maybe even over a couple of years. Then as they begin to feel more comfortable, this becomes rather intermittent and they may only call on you in times of stress. You feel that they are doing well when they do not call. Then, they have developed a relationship to you that has some substance and they have been allowed to say what they think and what they feel and what is really going on. This means that you expect parents early to voice a great many of the difficulties I mentioned—their own guilt, their rage, why did it happen to them.

On a block with young mothers, there is often competition about who got farthest with toilet training first. Of course, the mothers with the girls usually win. The boys are toilet trained later. This kind of competitive quality always exists, so a mother who feels that she has given birth to a child with a handicap, a defect, feels that she is really lost in this race. Do not expect a person just to ask you how to handle the situation and let it go at that. If the mother has a child that has been born very recently and she does not voice a lot of these other things, there is something missing. You should tell parents that mothers who have children with clefts have many other questions. If you have a counseling group that is going, that is available, it is very helpful if they join the group.

If you are in an area where there are not that many children then you should see the mother alone over a period of time and also see the father. You know how terrifying babies are to fathers; they do not know what to do with them. They are afraid to handle them or to hold them until they gradually begin to smile and to sit up; then they become acceptable. So you can imagine how terrifying a child with a handicap is to a father. He just does not know what to do with it most of the time. He is not able to manage it and he keeps away. This is why it is very important to bring the father in. Also, out of his need to deny his own involvement and his own fears, anytime there is some stress, the father can easily blame the mother because he has put 100 percent of the burden on her to handle the whole situation. So any failure is hers. Obviously, it is not his because he has unconsciously made the decision to divorce himself from the situation, so it cannot be his fault because he did not take the responsibility, and besides it is from the other side of the family, anyway.

There is another thing that I think is important. If you are in an area where there is not a team working, or if the parents have had the surgery done elsewhere, do not assume that they are being told a great deal, that they really understand it, that they know what is going on, and that they have had a chance to receive counseling. I never assume that, because often it has never happened. I think you should ask them what they have heard, what they have been told; what they think the future is; how they really felt when they had this child; and where they have been. If they say that they have talked to somebody, you should ask them how much have they talked, how long, and how often. This is true about any kind of counseling. I do a great deal of consultation for emotionally disturbed children and the first thing I ever ask anybody, whether it is from an agency or privately, is where they have been before, who they have talked to, what they have been told, and whether there was any treatment because sometimes they are just looking for another answer that is unavailable at the present time and I cannot help.

Sometimes they know nothing. But never assume that a person or a family who has had trouble has heard a great deal or heard a little. You know they have heard something, they have gotten involved somewhere, because a person, especially with a medical problem like a cleft, has gotten something somewhere. But you do not know what it is and you do not know how distorted it is and what they really know about the future. So I often ask what has happened and what they have been told for another reason—to avoid another trap. If you do not, they tell you everything and then you say, "Well, I think you should do this," and the mother says, "Well, we have tried that, but that has failed," and then you say, "Perhaps this would work." They say, "We have been told to do that, but that hasn't worked either." Then you get the message. She is out to fail and to get you to fail no matter what happens. You are just not going to win because she has a need to suffer and also to cripple you and possibly to cripple her child. You know the mother who is very long suffering, who is very masochistic; her rage and her feelings that are so sadistic have to be held in check so that she will go through the motions of doing the right thing, but you know that that has got to fail. But she has to say that she is doing it right and is altruistic. So I think you should always ask mothers and fathers what they have been told and whether they have carried it out and how they carried it out and what has happened.

A mother like this can be very pleasant, but you find after quite a period of time that you begin to get irritated with her and you wonder why. You know that you are mad at her because she is making you fail and you sense that you are not going to win; she is going to win the battle. A mother like this often is very depressed underneath because she is so angry and there is no outlet for her anger, for herself, for the child, for the doctor. It can go to extremes. There was once a mother who had a child with hemophilia, who decided to prove that the doctor and nurses did not really watch over him. When she went out for lunch one day, she took a roll of toilet paper and strung it around the crib of her little boy and when she came back and it was not broken, it was proof to her that nobody ever watched over her child, nobody ever looked at him, nobody ever cared for him; you can get quite paranoid, and she was. But these are extremes that you see.

I think that perhaps as a physician-psychiatrist, more as a physician, with malpractice judgments being what they are these days, you always have to ask people what they are doing; otherwise, you or the company might be out a million dollars. And no matter what you have heard of a physician's income, not many of us can afford that kind of judgment. But, more seriously, you want to extend help and we all do, but we should never fall into the trap that because your wishes are the best and this is what you want to do, that this is what is being accepted by the family. The family is a very complicated structure and all kinds of nonverbal nuances that are important for you to try to understand run through a family. If something does not ring true, you should ask more about it so that you have to extend yourself in terms of listening to what has been done, and then what the family expects from you, and what might be the limitations.

It is so important to leave the treatment open ended, especially with a child who has a handicap. You do not know what the final results are going to be. You can have a child with an excellent anatomic result who still is not speaking well because there is a need in the family to keep him crippled. The mother will still try to pinpoint some very superficial, subtle defect as the reason for the child not talking well, and this is not true, but she has a need to keep this child tied to her so that he should never change. One reason for this might be that once she has allowed him to separate, her main reason for being a mother and being accepted, and also a reason for her being able to get away with so much in terms of letting other duties go, is gone. Then she may have to do other things that are very difficult for her to do. I bring out many issues that sometimes do not occur to people during therapy because all mothers are mothers, you know, and obviously all mothers want to do the best they can. Consciously they do and unconsciously they do, too, but for other reasons that are very complicated in relation to their own desires. After all, a mother is a woman first, and she is not a wife first. She is an individual who is a mother first and that may have very little to do with all the other things that we talked about. This often makes therapists very uncomfortable. I am not talking about you as speech therapists, but people doing counseling and guidance. They do not like to get into this kind of situation that goes beyond support, advice, reeducation, environmental manipulation, and resources, because then they have to get into things that are personal. In the most difficult cases, you have got to get into the things that are more personal or you are never going to be able to help the child come to an adequate resolution of his problem because these are the things that are the resistances holding it back.

It may be that if you in the end are not able to devote

enough time to a certain family, you have to refer them to a child guidance clinic or a family therapy agency. I have often found in working with a child guidance clinic or consulting with agencies that they are very frightened of taking children who have handicaps, so it works both ways. Often people fall into the trap of thinking, "If he has a handicap, what can we do for him psychologically?" The answer is that they can do as much for him as they do for anybody else and sometimes more. There is a classic kind of example of children who are retarded who develop a psychosis. You might imagine that with a psychosis and a child who is mentally retarded the outlook is grim because he did not have that much to begin with. He was not equal with other children. But the truth is that most often the psychosis in children who are mentally retarded has an extremely good prognosis. The reason for it is that children who are retarded are extremely dependent on the environment. They are concrete, they must look to their parents or whoever is taking care of them. Often the reason that they have become psychotic temporarily is that there has been too much pressure, just direct pressure for achievement or for some other reason, or perhaps some catastrophe in the family and they cannot cope with it. As soon as you can alleviate the pressure or change the environment, you see this melt away very quickly.

Therefore, do not assume because there is a certain type of handicap that the outlook is less than what it would be with the child who has no handicap, though no physical disability must be better. And I can cite many, many examples of this. For example, a child who is now going to college somewhat handicapped because of a blood disease, who not only had to fight that but his parents telling him he should never go to college. It did not have to do with the illness entirely, but this just was not their style of life and he was just wasting his life and four years, and he is so crazy to do such a thing. But with counseling over the last three years, he has been able to fight this and grow up and separate. Which brings up another matter. When you are working with parents and you get into the areas beyond support, advice, reeducation, and getting resources for them, you should not expect them always to be thankful to you for discovering certain things and making them aware of the problems that they have. They do not like that. None of us like to have someone tell us what we do not like to hear and we know is right. It is sort of an injury to his own self-esteem. Eventually they will like you again, but you have to expect a certain amount of resistance and anger and resentment on the part of the parents when you are talking about an image of themselves that they know is there, but that they do not want to know is there. You know, it is like conveniently forgetting where you put something or conveniently forgetting a distasteful job that you should do.

All of this means that you have to be very tactful in approaching these things that are denied. You always have to give parents several alternatives; it is possible that they could feel this way; it would not be unusual if they would feel a certain way. You are not saying that they do, but they can be angry or resentful or worried about their capabilities, but at least they can think about it. And this kind of discussion does not occur in one session. It occurs over a period of time and you have to be available on an intermittent basis, often for a number of years.

Someone said once that the best way to have only therapeutic successes is to move every three years. Then you do not have the people coming back to you. And it is true. You build up a case load after a while and that stays with you; as long as you stay there, they are going to be around to show you that you are not quite perfect. Everybody who does therapy of any sort has a feeling of hoping to undo something and make people perfect. Learning to do therapy, no matter what kind of therapy, has to do with learning to live with less than perfect results in many people, which basically is learning to live with the human condition that we are all less than perfect, both emotionally and physically, and that in the end a handicap does not have to be demobilizing or permanent on any level at all.

I don't think that people, in general, very quickly can accept a deformity of any sort. It is too frightening. And as I have emphasized throughout this session, fear is the initial reaction. People with seizures used to be, as you know, banned from the village because to see someone having seizures is so terrifying; either you banned them or you made them a priest. And this is the reaction of most people to anything that is very deviant. You either exalt them or you kick them out or kill them. And everybody still reacts in the same way, no matter what is said about differences in human beings. The initial reaction is one of terror. And you do not tell this to everybody; you do not hold this as great knowledge. It is just something that exists. Then very quickly a person recovers and does what he can. This is what anybody doing therapy attempts to do and understands the source of his own fears.

If you understand the source of your own concerns, you can always understand the source of concern that the parents have and the child will have. And I am sure that all of you get results very quickly. Results may come over a year, two years, three years with painstaking work, while the emotional aspects of working with the parents of the children who have clefts, then the children themselves, are quiescent; and then you might have a period of stress because the child finds it difficult to adjust in a new situation; or the child's developmental level, or what he is doing, or where he is going may arouse feelings in the parent that they did not have at the earlier time because they just were well adapted to what he was doing then.

So treatment often is an intermittent thing over a period of years and certainly I would advocate early working with groups of parents as a way to help them feel a common bond to find many answers and to feel that they are not alone and isolated and that there are many things that they can understand from others who have had the same experience. You as the leader can help them a great deal.

Chapter 7

THE ROLE OF THE PEDIATRICIAN
IN CLEFT PALATE MANAGEMENT

Robert Chesky

THE PROBLEMS of the cleft palate child are complex and decisions about one area often get into considerations that involve another area of expertness. It is quite obvious that the team approach, whether it is organized on a formal basis or is an informal group of people who work separately but who have close ties with each other, means a great deal. And I think, from what I can understand about it, that you do not want to entrust the child to the occasional practitioner. Therefore, I want to discuss the way in which the cleft palate team works in the state of Michigan.

I do not know a lot about the statewide situation. In Detroit, there are cleft palate teams at Children's Hospital; there is a team at Sinai Hospital. In Ann Arbor, there are groups working out of both the University and St. Joseph's Hospital that work along some of the lines that I talked about in terms of team approach. The efforts at Children's— I do not know about Sinai—are aided by the State Health Department. Cleft palate teams, for the most part, are set up under the auspices of the State Health Department and are aided by funds available from the State Health Department via Crippled Children's funds. Crippled Children's programs nationwide started forty to fifty years ago and were aimed at, via Washington and state matching programs, health programs for orthopedically handicapped children. Probably, earlier impetus was related to the period when polio was the main consideration. These programs have since broadened and the definition of crippled children has expanded to the point where chronic handicapping conditions of many kinds are included in the Crippled Children's program. Children with these handicaps are aided by the formation of clinics, like the cleft palate clinics, or epilepsy clinics, or orthopedically handicapped clinics, and so on, through the state. The State Health Department will pay the bills for people that cannot afford these kinds of treatments on a private basis, and finances are a substantial consideration in the getting of all this complex variety of specialists to give care to a child; very few people can afford that kind of thing on a private basis. So if you are in Detroit or eastern Michigan, I think I pointed out several places. If you are out of state, I am sure that the State Health Department would be a ready source of information about the closest cleft palate team available to wherever you live.

The Health Department also imposes certain quality controls in this regard. If they are going to support and pay for the services rendered by a cleft palate team, they require that the plastic surgeon be a Board-certified plastic surgeon with experience in this area, and they will not pay for the services of other kinds. If you try this route, the state of Michigan has imposed certain quality controls on the whole business and has insured that the general practitioner up in Manistee is not getting paid for doing cleft palate and cleft lip repairs by the Commission. The Commission has confined the business to people who are experienced at it; I think that is a good thing. So, the State Health Department would be the best source of information for you about resources in this regard for children whom you do not think are getting proper medical care via your local programs, and you should keep this in mind here in Michigan.

Let us consider the immediate impact of the birth of a cleft palate child. Management of the parent, particularly immediately upon birth of this child, in light of the fact that the mother suffers a certain amount of separation depression in most cases following the birth of a normal child anyhow, is quite compounded with this kind of very asocial birth, and so on. How, right from the moment of birth, do the obstetrician and the pediatrician, having seen the child within the first several hours of life, start to manage the parental reaction and the parental handling of the child? They must be thinking now of the parents' immediate reaction, telling how the parents in three or four days are going to feel being totally responsible for the care of the child and maybe have some ambivalence about it. With all these parameters that are involved, how do the doctors get the parent involved, to start looking realistically? The question really is how *should* they?

I think a lot of things are done that should not be done in this regard. I have seen, in the course of a few years in pediatrics, several things that I would think you know as being pretty horrendous examples of how they do it. I recall very vividly a woman who was thirty-eight years old and unmarried, who got pregnant by a man she refused to name and had her first child illigitimately some place out in the western part of the state and came back to Detroit to live with her parents. The child had a cleft palate and she presented the child when it was ten or twelve days old, as I recall it. The child, almost literally, had never gotten a drop to eat up to that point; had lost a pound or a pound and a half. Nobody had ever told her about the defect before she went home from the hospital. I think they told her the day she went home that the child had a cleft palate and they had given her no feeding instructions whatsoever about it or how to handle it. This just happened last year. We rounded up a nurse who had been on the nursery and knew a great deal about feeding cleft palate kids and sat her down with the lady and rounded up some bottles. We use a lamb's nipple frequently at Children's. This is not a nationwide thing. There are all kinds of devices you use to feed these kids, but the lamb's nipple is probably long enough and has a kind of a tapering shape with a big round end and big hole in it. It goes way back into the mouth and almost drips the stuff down the gullet, as it were, with very little sucking. Feeding is mainly a milking action and a compression by the mouth, rather than a suck for the cleft palate child. Well, we taught her how to feed the baby, and as a result, with just that simple handling of that one problem, she thinks Children's Hospital has nothing but great people there. She had not received that much consideration in the previous hospital.

I recall another case where the cleft palate was entirely missed. The child had a complete cleft—no palate at all, practically, and the mother did very well with the child without the problem ever even being discovered; amazingly enough, she came in because the child would occasionally lose milk from his nose and she wanted to know why. Imagine my amazement when I looked in the mouth!

With an obviously deformed child, and here we are talking about a child with a bad cleft lip mainly, I am sure the obstetrician would try in some way to whiz the baby out of the delivery room on some pretext or other until the mother is in a state where she could be better informed about the child. This delay in the mother's seeing the child should not be a long one; if it is prolonged too much, fantasy becomes worse than reality. And the mother may imagine she has a mongoloid, she has a child without any arms or legs, or a variety of things which are far worse than what is really the case.

So, whoever is in charge, whether it be the obstetrician or the pediatrician, depending upon who has the best rapport with the family, should break the news. Often, the father is told first and is allowed to compose himself. Then, the father and the physician involved tell the mother. This is true of a variety of defects, not just cleft lip and cleft palate. There is a horrifying aspect to it, something should be done to cushion the shock; the mother should not be confronted with this immediately after birth, when she is in no shape after hours and hours of labor to withstand much; but it should not be delayed.

Some people cover up cleft lips with a piece of tape or a piece of cotton and a piece of tape or something like this when they show the mother the child for the first time. Cleft palate is not so much a problem because, as I said earlier, the defect does not give a grotesque appearance to the child; it is not obvious. Here the problem is mainly some instruction in feeding before the child leaves the hospital if it is a cleft palate alone. If it is a cleft palate and lip or cleft lip alone, the child may stay in the hospital until the operation is done. And this is thought by many to build a better relationship, because the mother does not have to deal with the child, feed it, take care of it day and night when he is obviously deformed. It is much better psychologically to have her take the baby home after the operation is done. That is the standard, current way of handling it.

QUESTION: Can a child be moved from one hospital to another for surgery?

ANSWER: Yes. I think if operative surgery were contemplated early with a newborn, most surgeons would want a hospital where anesthesia is customarily given to small infants and that usually means the Children's Hospital or a hospital with a large pediatric service. The anesthesia is an important part of the rest of the surgery. As far as the postoperative nursing care is concerned, too, there are specialized facets of that which require a hospital that is accustomed to dealing with a child. For example, devices are applied to the face to save the repair of the lip and to reduce the tension on the incision and the closure. If a spring device is attached to the cheeks, it must stay on. The child's arms are pinned to his sides so that he cannot get his fists up to his mouth and break down this very delicate incision or repair line. Feeding is different; he can not be allowed to suck very soon after. There cannot be any great tension on the mouth very soon after surgery. So the nursing care is specialized, too.

I think all of these things will mitigate in favor of Children's Hospital or a place where this kind of surgery and nursing is done. As a matter of fact, if my baby were involved I would want it done at Children's Hospital or a place that did a lot of children's surgery or infant surgery. Infant surgery is not all that common. No general hospital in Manistee is going to do very much of it.

QUESTION: Because of the parents' reaction to this when they first see the child, can you relate any generalization that you found that works, a certain psychology that works, in informing the parents that they have a cleft palate child? Are there any generalizations that you can make? How do you approach the parents?

ANSWER: I think the principal approach that I would use is to be factual without being brutal. I mean you cannot walk in and say you have cancer, or you cannot walk in and say your child has cleft palate, and then leave. You have to leave the people with something in the way of a realistic picture and hope for the future. The time to talk about the future of the child with cleft lip or cleft palate is when you go in to inform the parents. And you ought to try to leave them something of a picture of what is available to the child and the type of problem that he is going to have in facing it. I have not done this very much with cleft palate, but I have found it to be very beneficial with a number of things. For example, when I pick up a murmur that I know is representative of an organic heart disease, I tell the parents. I tell them I am sorry I have to tell them this, but I think they have to know and will have to face it together now. I then explain to them what a heart murmur is and what it means; how some heart murmurs mean organic heart disease, some do not; I think this means heart disease; this may mean that it has to be corrected by surgery; it may not be correctable. I think it is one or the other. But I am not competent to make the final decision. Here is how this decision is made. We go through this, this, and this diagnostic procedure. We do it at particular times. What are the reasons for doing this diagnostic procedure? What about surgery; when is that done? In general, what is going to happen to the child for some years to come, in a general way, without so much data that it is confusing?

QUESTION: Do you advocate taping up the lip to make the child more attractive cosmetically to the parents before you show them?

ANSWER: Well, I have not really thought about it. I just might, depending upon how grotesque it is, I suppose. If it is a complete bilateral cleft, it would depend on how bad the defect was.

Doctor Falk comments: It seems to me that you could come up with any number of kids that you could not hide behind a piece of gauze or a piece of tape; you get into some children with damage to the premaxilla, and the unusual deformity that results, and so it is pretty hard to hide. You might minimize appearance at first until the mother has handled this child a couple of times and then slowly take away the bandage and introduce her to what it really looks like underneath. It seems to be a temporary thing, at best. Hopefully the pediatrician knows the parents before this birth and knows that the parent has other children, to get a feel of the general emotional makeup of the mother. I think the father will tend to hide behind his facade of masculinity, anyhow, and the mother is really the one you have to be concerned about. However, I do not think you should sell the father short when you know that there are cases right here in Detroit where the father has deserted the family upon the birth. But it is the mother who is really going to have the chief role in this even if the father has a pretty good attitude. And so she is really the one you will have to deal with.

DR. CHESKY: I do not think you can delay the truth very long; it is just not wise. This is our worst problem. I think that there are lots of ways of telling the truth. Physicians just instinctively pick them up, just as school teachers, politicians,

and everybody else does. It is a little hard to generalize on
the basis that people have different personalities. It has somewhat to do with my personality. Do you explain to the parents
the correct way the velum should work? No, I do not. I just
have not had that much to do with that. When I had my
training and my experience here, the plastic surgeon took over
the lip repair at the newborn period and the pediatrician was
pretty well excluded from the whole business. Now I think
that as a practicing pediatrician, I will probably be considerably
more involved in that. I think somebody ought to explain it.
I think that shows something of the virtue of the team approach. All of us get our blinders on and a plastic surgeon
that thinks that once he has repaired the thing, the job is
done, is going to be sadly mistaken. If we do not look at the
end results of either cosmesis or speech, we are missing the
boat.

The topic has to do with the pediatrician's approach to
cleft palate and pediatric care of cleft palate and the patient.
In effect, I will say a little more about this in detail later on.
I do not think a pediatrician should be considered an expert
on cleft palate any more than he should be an expert on a
number of diseases that involve a variety of specialists who
know more about individual facets of the thing than the pediatrician does. The pediatrician is a generalist and his object
in the cleft palate program, on the cleft palate team, is to
provide a cohesive force and a member who understands basically what the problems are in all the fields. Often in various
types of clinic arrangements, he acts as a mediator between
the varying groups and a communicator with parents. So my
approach is that of a generalist, not of a person who has a
particular career interest in cleft palate or could be logically
considered to be a real specialist in that area. Hence, I think
you ought to take what I say with a grain of salt, in that
when I deal with things that other people know more about,
do you want to listen to the other people or compare what I
say with what they say? Think about it.

I want to begin by placing some emphasis on the importance of cleft palate as a pediatric and public health problem and to do so, I can think of no better way than to talk something about the statistics involved. Cleft palate is one of the most common congenital anomalies of childhood and occurs approximately once in every eight hundred births. When you consider the millions of births per year in the United States, you can really appreciate that we are producing literally thousands of children with variations of cleft lip and palate each year. Of this group, almost fifty percent have both cleft lips and palates. About 25 percent have either cleft lips alone or cleft palate alone. About 10 percent of the children have other anomalies of varying degrees and magnitude and I will mention some of them briefly as we go along. I think the important statistic to think about here is that 90 percent of the children with cleft lip and palate have no other abnormality or defect and should be considered to be, in that respect, normal until proven otherwise by the parent or by the teacher who encounters them in school. I think the statistics alone emphasize the importance of the problem.

Another way of looking at the problem is to consider the consequences of poor treatment, management, and habilitation. It is readily appreciable that a cosmetic defect of this sort imposes real psychological strains on both the individual who is affected with the problem and upon the family that is confronted with it. The defective speech that may develop from improper repair of palate defects or lip defects imposes throughout life a burden that may be crippling. You may or may not appreciate that defective hearing is often an accompaniment of cleft palate disorders, and improper handling of this defect may also be a lifelong crippling proposition. The problem of malocclusion and absence of teeth from a cosmetic and functional speech standpoint requires the utmost care and handling and the consequences of improper management in that regard are important. You can readily appreciate that all of these things have a great deal to do with educability and later employability of the child. Hence, a problem of this magnitude statistically and with so many ways to go wrong must give us all cause, as far as proper handling is concerned, as a major public health problem.

Next, I would like to say something about cause. A great deal is known other than that over 20 percent of these children are from families in which a story of cleft palate or harelip or both are involved. So you know heredity is of great importance in a substantial number of cases, perhaps 20 or 25 percent. For the other 75 percent, we know of no cause although we can speculate on the basis of experiments with various forms of experimental animals that environmental disorders in the first three months of life may be important. We do know that certain animals consistently reproduce litters with cleft palate or lips or both when certain vitamins are withheld from the mother. We do know that adding certain substances to the diet—for example, massive amounts of cortisone—can lead to cleft lip and palate in experimental animals, and other unusual stresses have been contrived and have consistently led to cleft lip and palate in experimental animals. These situations are rarely reproduced in adult humans who are pregnant, but the evidence, such as it is, would indicate that environment does affect this. Obviously, like any other anomaly, in the overwhelming majority of which the causes are unknown, we have to assume that there are factors at work of that sort that have yet to be elucidated.

Basically, cleft lip and palate represent a failure of fusion of embryologically separate parts, and a whole wide spectrum of congenital anomalies are of this sort. The structures involved are separate structures at early points of human development and fail to unite as they normally would between the third and twelfth weeks of gestational life and leave the child with the resulting deformity. There is some evidence that failure of union of the lip fragments is a result of events prior to the seventh week and the palate union involves a later period—eighth to the twelfth week.

The lip and palate deformities are of varying severity and may range in the case of the lip from a small cleft on one side that involves the vermilion border of the lip all the way to clefts ascending all the way to the floor of the nose and involving the nostril. The lip defects, of course, may be on one side or on both sides and, as I stated, may be complete or incomplete depending on where they go from and how far they go up the lip. The complete clefts of the lip may or may not involve abnormalities of the ridged gum that we know, the alveolar ridge, from which the teeth emerge.

The complete lip cleft may involve dental ridge involution, lack of development of the alveolar ridge; it may involve extra, absent, or deformed teeth. The cartilage of the nose and the lateral portion of the nose may be involved, or may be deformed or displaced, leading to further cosmetic problems in terms of correction. In bilateral complete cleft lips, the columella, or the portion of the nose which leads from the tip to the upper portion of the lip, may be very deficient and may present major problems in terms of plastic repair.

On the other hand, cleft palates may involve merely a notch and may be extremely variable in extent, just like lips; they may involve only a notch in the uvula, or the little piece of tissue that hangs down off the soft palate. It may go all the way up the entire front of the mouth and, as I am sure you are aware, the clefts may only involve bone without involving soft tissue *and* bone. This represents some occasional cause of nasal speech—cleft palate speech without an obvious physical deformity.

Commonly you have encountered another associated anomaly that we see fairly often—the so-called Pierre Robin syndrome. Although Robin did not write the original description of the problem, he elucidated and clarified it to such an extent that his name became attached to it. The Pierre Robin syndrome is cleft palate associated with a very small mandible or jaw. Either because of the extremely small lower jaw, the so-called "Andy Gump" lower jaw, or because of abnormalities of relative muscle strength and relative pulls on the position of the tongue, the tongue drops back into the oral pharynx and interferes with feeding and breathing. This is one of the truly life-threatening states associated with cleft palate, and because of the position of the tongue and its interference with the airway of the child, these children are handled in a variety of ways which I will go into later. As an associated anomaly, it is perhaps one you ought to be aware of when you see a child with a cleft palate problem and a small jaw. In time, the survivors, I would say most of them that we see in the clinic, develop normal mandibles and very few persist in having small lower jaws until school age when you would be likely to see them. I cannot quote statistics, but there are a few children that continue to have small jaws. I was rather impressed by that. Before I came to cleft palate clinic, I saw most of them at birth when they are in real trouble and the children really look deformed in a major way. However, when you see them later on within the age group you see how well their jaws have grown. At Children's Hospital here the common practice was to perform a tracheotomy on these children if they were in major difficulty and then get the tube out as soon as the jaw achieved sufficient size to support the tongue and keep it away from the back of the throat. It is usually a successful approach. Doctor McEvitt has, I believe, compiled his series of sixty of these children and handling of them and his success rate is very good as compared to the world literature on this subject. Many of the children die. We had a few deaths, mainly from children who came in virtually moribund to Children's.

I would like to discuss the team approach to cleft palate work and analyze what the members of the team do, as well as the function of the medical team and the ancillary team that supports it. The development of modern surgical techniques led to the ability to repair cleft lips and cleft palates long before the operative procedures were well defined and before consistent good results could be achieved. And as children began to survive their defect and live to adult life, it became apparent the long-term result of therapy was far from what might be desirable in terms of functional speech and cosmetic repair. The complexity of the problem became apparent and the work of a number of specialists was necessary to properly handle the problem. This has been perhaps the major development, as I understand it, in the history of cleft palate work from a medical standpoint in the last twenty or twenty-five years. It is an approach that is not unusual nowadays in handling a variety of complicated problems. The pattern of multiple specialists working together in a group has obvious merit in a number of different fields.

I will just go on by discussing the composition of the team and what the individual members of the group do, as I understand it and as I have experienced it here in Detroit. As I suggested earlier, the function of a pediatrician is that of general health supervision of the children and general health advice to the parent of the child with cleft palate. A major portion of this, I think, is anticipatory guidance in terms of the psychological problems that the child will encounter as the time passes. This is certainly true if the pediatrician has the proper setting and time to give to the patients and time to get to know the families. Feeding problems are major problems early in life and this is especially true with the child with cleft palate. In other places, the pediatrician is often the head of the cleft palate team and as such, serves as a coordinator and interpreter of advice of more specialized individuals. In the case of the organization of the teams here, the plastic surgeons head the teams and provide essentially the same service of coordinating the results from the various specialists, making recommendations, and interpreting to the parents. The pediatrician is another member of the team whose advice is taken when it seems desirable and necessary. I think either way works all right, depending on the personalities involved. The plastic surgeon perhaps is always one of the key members of the team. It is his job to decide what surgical procedures to use and when to use them. These procedures are by no means cut and dried. They are not universally agreed upon and, will vary according to the skill of the surgeon, his training, and the kind of procedures he is used to doing. I think that it is obvious that the ultimate long-term result in many of these cases is the result of the skill and experience of the plastics man who is ultimately responsible for these kinds of decisions.

The lip surgery and the timing of lip closure in cases of either cleft lip alone or lip and palate is usually quite early. By early, I mean somewhere between forty-eight hours and eight weeks of age, usually in the area of about a month to six weeks. Usually nobody will operate on a premature child. They will probably wait until the child weighs about six pounds, until he is eating and gaining weight reasonably well and is in a decent state of fluid balance and metabolic balance before surgery is undertaken. Hence, the risk of surgery is reduced by all of these measures. The closure of the lip at an early stage is extremely important from a psychological standpoint. There is great difficulty in the mother's accepting a child with a deformity as obvious as a cleft lip, depending, of course, upon how extensive the cleft is. Let us assume that it is a major cleft or a complete one and it has been deemed appropriate to get this repair done even before the child goes home from the hospital so that the relationship between the mother and the child will not be impaired by the presence of such an obvious defect at such an early date, at such an early and crucial time in the relationship between the two.

The timing of the primary palatal repair in cases of cleft palate is considerably later, principally because growth and development of the structures involved in closure are impaired by a very early operation in comparison with the cleft lip. And practices vary across the country, but the time may be as early as a year, or may be extended to as late as five years, depending on the anatomic factors and tissues involved and the judgments of the cleft palate team as to how efficacious prostheses are in taking care of the problems of the cleft palate part of the surgery. Here in Detroit, the palates are closed fairly shortly after a year; or at least a primary closure is attempted. Some closures are incomplete and further operations as well as prostheses may be necessary to tide the child over until the infinity of problems can be handled. The principal psychological reason for early closure would be to get the child done before speech development has been impaired and before he has learned faulty speech habits due to the cleft. I am sure across the country, as in any field, the result will vary according to competence of the surgeon, the individual technique involved, and the individual surgical procedure involved; so it is very difficult to generalize. And I think, too, that our long-term follow-ups are such that it is hard to generalize validly and scientifically. Only with the development of cleft palate teams are we getting something like the kind of follow-up that we need to determine our results.

Continuing to talk about plastic surgery, other procedures are frequently necessary. As I have implied, the kids with Pierre Robin syndrome may be required to have a tracheotomy as a life-saving technique. Surgical procedures for keeping the tongue out of the way have been fantastically variable around the world. Some people put a stitch through the tongue and tie it around the mandible to hold the tongue forward. Some people have rigged devices to hook the stitch to a rubber band sort of arrangement, anchored high in the air so that the tongue is pulled up out of the throat and the airway kept free. I read about one courageous man who reported wrapping the back of the child's head in something very tight and suspending the head so that the tongue would hang forward and he only lost the scalp in two out of three cases and decided that that was not a very good procedure. I think he had a lot of courage to report it. This particular problem led to a lot of very imaginative approaches.

Revisions of both the lip and nose are frequent after the primary repair and are usually done when the child is older. Then there is more tissue to work with and further growth of the underlying bony structures will not damage the ultimate result. As I suggested earlier, palatal closures may not be complete and further operations are necessary. The timing needs to be decided upon for complete closures of the palate or to close the fistulas involved in the palate.

In summary, as far as the factors involved in the plastic surgery here in terms of timing and procedures and selection of procedures, I think we have to consider cosmetic result and the psychological factors involved in prolonging surgery. We also have to consider the ultimate speech result and psychological factors associated with poor speech development. This has to be weighed in the balance; we have to weigh selection of surgical procedures and the effect of surgery on the underlying bony structures, in particular the parts of these bony structures from which growth takes place. The size of the defect and the available tissue to redo the repairs has to be considered. This often points toward later surgery because the growth of tissues sometimes makes it an easier proposition to work with. We have to consider the prevention of ear infections and accumulations of fluid that are so common in this disorder which often mitigate in favor of urgent, early surgery and early closure of clefts. In deciding about the surgery, you have to consider what other measures are available to handle the problems that you have in case you do not do surgery; for example, the prostheses that could be provided to aid in the development of normal speech or to close the palate.

So much for the surgical aspects. Cleft palate teams at Children's and most places have a prosthodontist as an integral part of the team. His line of work is palatal prostheses either before the primary repair or, as I suggested, sometimes after the primary repair pending complete closure. These prostheses may be considered as aids in developing normal speech and may be important in tiding the patient over till his physical condition permits surgery. For example, some children fail to thrive on their feeding procedures. I think I have run into a fair percentage of cases at Children's that were really quite dwarfed early in life by their feeding problems imposed by the cleft palate. Here, again, you do not want to close the palate until you have a child big enough to operate on. Hence the prosthesis may be necessary to tide a child like that over until his physical condition permits surgery. Some people think that the prosthetic devices applied at something like ages two to three, prior to any surgical repair, help to develop the soft palate and the pharyngeal muscles so that the later definitive operation to close the palate may result in better speech than in the cases that were operated on earlier without the prosthodontic device. Again, I think that this is something that varies from center to center. The prosthodontist may also be involved in providing artificial dentures where needed. This is most important in complete clefts involving both sides of the mouth, that is, complete cleft lips and palate on both sides. When the problem is of the premaxilla, the most frontal portion of the bony structures in this area, dental problems are at their maximum.

The orthodontist is another essential member of the team, and his principal task is to provide the best possible dental arch for chewing and for speech. He is often working in the presence of absent teeth, impacted teeth, misplaced teeth, or extra teeth. The orthodontist's work is somewhat different in cleft palate in that he is not only moving teeth about and trying to get them into proper position to form a decent arch for speech and for chewing but he is also involved in attempting to position the alveolar ridge and the premaxillary fragments properly.

I wonder if the pediatricians are not going to go the way of dentists with all these subspecialties in dentistry—I can hardly keep track any more and it is getting as complicated as this. Anyway, just the plain, ordinary dentist is often a member of the cleft palate team and his job is important because dental decay is more of a factor in these children than in normal children, because the position of their teeth often prevents them from getting the natural cleansing actions of saliva, the tongue, the gums, the insides of the cheeks, and so on. So maintenance of teeth is often necessary, since they provide anchors for prostheses or a means of straightening other defective or malformed teeth. Thus it is very important to keep all the teeth. Also, maintenance of all the teeth is important for the proper growth of the jaws. Hence, just simple prevention of decay and repair of decayed teeth and keeping these in the mouth so that they can be utilized for other purposes, or to maintain proper growth of the jaw is of great importance.

I do not think I need to talk to you about the importance of speech training in this regard. I do not know a lot about it, compared to what you do. It would seem to me that without normal speech, half of the job is not done with the child with cleft lip and palate. And the other half, perhaps, would be the ultimate cosmetic result. Either absence of normal speech or absence of relatively normal appearance, I think, is a life-crippling proposition and the speech work, like the other work, should be undertaken early and monitored just as frequently and carefully as the physical repair of the defects.

The ear, nose and throat man and the audiologist, whose concern is with hearing, are other vital members of the team. Most data show that upwards of 25 percent of these cases have significant impairments of hearing; ear infections are frequent, possibly due to the lack of any separation between the nasopharynx and entry of fluid into the eustachian tube which leads to the middle ear. We found this to be a problem very early in life, rather frequently, even in the first year, and adenoidectomies have been performed in the first year in an attempt to promote drainage from the eustachian tubes and to keep them open. Later on, as infection takes place, not only is vigorous antibiotic treatment utilized but so are procedures such as myringotomy, where the eardrum is punctured and fluid or pus let out, or tubes are placed in the middle ear to promote the constant drainage of fluid. Often other necessary ancillary procedures are performed. And so in our clinic here, and I think in most places, the ENT and audiology people are vital members of the team.

Other teams use social workers, public health nurses, and members of the psychiatric profession, either clinical psychologists or psychiatrists, as either members of the team or consultants. I read about one team that routinely refers all of its adolescent patients with cleft lip and palate problems to the psychiatric service because of the incidence of problems with their adjustment to their defect at this age. As all of you know, adolescence is an extremely stormy time and in pediatrics we find it true that this is the time of life when conformity and lack of major differences between the child and his peer group are of primary importance. This is the time when uniforms and fads are most prevalent and when individual differences between children are tolerated least well by the children themselves. And this is a time when the child with an obvious physical defect will be most uncomfortable. Just as a sidelight, we find the same thing true with our teenage diabetics; there is not one of them who does not at some point in his adolescence rebel against his disease and refuse to control his diet and his insulin therapy and goes way off the deep end in terms of his balance and ends up in real trouble. Some children do it repeatedly until they learn to make the adjustment to live with their disease, and I think those are quite possibly some of the same factors that are at work in cleft palate. Obviously, the defect sets the child apart and makes him different in some way that he can not tolerate at this time of his life.

Perhaps I should conclude this by saying something about the usual parental reactions to these children. I think that some of this has importance to you as teachers and therapists and you could probably tell stories that will illustrate these points as well as I can. In the psychiatric sense, the reaction to the birth of a defective child in the case of cleft palate, and other defects as well, is one of grief and mourning. What has been lost is the perfect baby that was dreamed about and anticipated and in its place there is a defective child, which is a surprise, a shock, a proof to the mother of her own inadequacy of producing children. This period of shock and grief is followed by a period of mourning, and all kinds of things take place in this period which are abnormal and need to be handled and understood if the mother, and eventually the father, too, are ultimately to be guided to the point where they can make a realistic appraisal of the situation and take a realistic approach to the whole prospect. All manner of fantasies are involved during this period of mourning. Physicians are often confronted by the fact that they are blamed, or the obstetrician is blamed, for whatever went wrong to produce this situation. And since we do not know what went wrong in the overwhelming majority of times, at least 75 percent of the time we do not know, this makes fantasizing all the easier. Use of x-rays in early pregnancy or blood transfusions in early pregnancy may be blamed for the problem. I read about one mother who blamed the fact that she had had two cleft palate children on the fact that her mother had not given her enough vitamins when she was a girl.

People are ashamed of their children, especially if they have the lip; the child with the cleft palate can be presented as a normal baby and shown to people in the same way that a normal baby could be and there is not quite the same situation as with the child with an obvious lip deformity. I read about two mothers that thought people would suspect that they had attempted abortion on themselves because their children had been born with cleft lips or palates and, hence, this led to major shame about displaying the child in public or even acknowledging the child. The fantasizing may be wholly demented and bizarre. One woman blamed her husband's cough which kept her awake at night for the problem. Another woman blamed her husband's demanding job that kept him away from home all of the time and left all of the work to her as the cause of the whole problem. All of these are things that may occur in the period immediately following the birth of the child when the mother's mind may run wild in this period of grief and mourning.

I think we are all appreciative enough of modern psychiatry to know how much emphasis is placed on feeding and mothering and affection in the early months of life in terms of the ultimate mental health of the child. And here we have a situation where a child is forbidden the nipple by some groups of cleft palate and harelip teams; is fed with a syringe, a dropper; often it is recommended that he be in an erect position which makes cuddling of the child difficult during feeding. If he has a cleft palate, he has substantial amounts coming out the nose. All in all, feeding, which is the most important early relationship between the mother and the child, is impaired and is rarely a relaxed, easy experience for the mother. The whole business may be so severely impaired that real problems may make it a wholly displeasurable experience. I think you can appreciate the psychological effects—that this might affect her image of herself as a mother—as a competent mother.

As time passes with these children and feeding problems become more resolved, parental reactions and anxieties are present whether they are admitted or not and center around a variety of factors. Their tooth eruption is often irregular and delayed. Many of these children are excessive droolers. When they start to vocalize in the last six months of the first year, they seem to do so less and it is often more monotonous than normal children. Many people think that their general speech is delayed, thus rearing a source of anxiety with the parents. Lurking behind all of these differences between the cleft palate child and the normal child is the suspicion that is very difficult to lay to rest in many parents—that the child is defective in more than just this way, that he is a monster, a retarded child; he has many more defects that the stupid doctors have not uncovered yet. Another, perhaps opposite, pendulum to this sort of reaction is the one that once the period of grief and mourning is over, the parent will refuse to admit to any differences between this child and a normal child and will ignore deviations that are present that need to be realistically encountered.

In short, you can conclude that the parent needs reassurance from the start and needs to be guided toward a realistic approach to the problem. A number of defense mechanisms have to be combatted in order to get the parent to arrive at a reasonable, rational, realistic approach. And this is one of the importances of a pediatrician or a generalist, or some member of the team who can act as one, in interpreting and anticipating problems of this sort that are sure to arise.

Perhaps the most difficult thing for the parent to bear in this kind of situation, the thing that can perhaps harm the whole business, is the physician's unwillingness to tell the truth and take the time to explain things rather than hiding them or assuring that he knows best—that the parent does not need information, so long as they follow him.

Chapter 8

DENTAL AND PROSTHETIC
MANAGEMENT OF CLEFT
LIP AND PALATE

K. W. Sproule and E. P. Hawthorne

Doctor Sproule: Prosthetics has been my field for the past forty years, and I became interested in the cleft palate child because of my sister who was afflicted by this same thing. So, it has been more of a hobby. When I started in, it was strictly by trial and error. And, as I might say, a good bit of it even today is by trial and error and correcting mistakes that we make as we go along.

Prosthetics is the replacement of the tissues of the mouth and the pharynx by mechanical means. This includes the teeth and hard and soft palate. For the cleft lip and palate child, this begins at the age of about three days and continues as the child develops, using interim appliances when necessary, to an age when growth stops at approximately eighteen to twenty years of age. At this time, a final appliance is made.

Our work is accomplished by means of different types of appliances. In the infant, the appliance used is made of silastic and is purely removable, fitting into the palatal cleft. This type will be gone into much more fully by Doctor Hawthorne, giving the reasons why it is used and what is accomplished.

Note: Throughout this chapter, the authors refer to slides which were shown at the Institute but which are now unavailable.

143

During the years of growth, transitional appliances must be constructed at such times as growth dictates. This is to allow for the eruption of teeth and still cover the defects. It also supplies necessary teeth to assist in speech and aesthetics. These appliances are also usually removable. The final appliance can be fixed, fixed-removable, removable using clasps, removable using fixed precision attachments, and removable using clasp precision attachments only, or any combination of the above. Also, a full denture may be used. The design of the case dictates which type should be used to give the best results.

In the construction of these appliances, each case must be studied very carefully, taking into consideration aesthetics, mastication, speech, and the type of construction which will function best for the particular individual.

In the study of each case, a complete oral examination is made, including visual oral examination and a complete x-ray study. Then, impressions are taken of both the upper and lower arches, models are made and jaw relations taken. These are transferred to an articulator. An articulator, in our work, is an instrument that we use to produce the movements of the jaws. At this time, decisions are made as to which teeth are nonusable and which teeth can be salvaged. Let me say here that some of these mouths have such a conglomeration of teeth and the orthodontist has found it impossible to get them anywhere near alignment, that it is necessary to remove many of them to make any kind of an appliance. These decisions made, we then remove the nonusable teeth from our models and proceed to design and plan whether it is to be fixed, fixed-removable, or removable, or which combination; and which teeth will support the appliances. And I will say here that we use full crowns on all supporting teeth.

Our plans are then discussed with the patient and the parents, and if they are agreeable, extractions are done and the mouth is allowed to heal for from about ten to fourteen days. New impressions are taken, models are poured, and jaw relations are made and mounted again on an articulator. From these new models we make a transitional appliance using plastic teeth and a plastic base, covering any fistula, contouring the palatal area, and setting the teeth in position for the aesthetics and speech. The anterior teeth should be placed in such a position that for the /f/ and /v/ sounds the lower lip touches the incisal edges of the upper teeth; enough free space exists for the child to be able to produce the *th* sounds; checks are made on the sibilant sounds, and, if necessary, the position of anterior teeth is changed and the palatal area is recontoured. If difficulty still persists, a thickening of the palatal base in the area of the tuberosities is made so that the airstream can be directed over the upper surface of the tongue.

With this appliance in place, the patient is sent back to the speech therapist for examination and instruction. These transitional appliances are worn for about four months to allow complete healing of the maxilla. This allows time for the patient to accomodate himself or herself to the appliance and also for us to know what changes should be made to improve it.

When healing has been completed, the work starts all over again. The supporting teeth are crowned and brought into occlusion. Impressions, models, and jaw relations are taken and transferred to the articulator. The final appliance will have a metal base and be contoured similar to the interim appliance and have clasps and attachments as were planned in the original design. The teeth are set up in wax so that any change can be made, and when they are in satisfactory position and the anterior palatal area is contoured, these are processed into plastic. When the patient has worn the appliance for about ten days, he returns to the speech therapist for final examination and instruction.

This procedure is strictly for the work anterior to the soft palate. However, if the patient has a short, immobile soft palate and cannot effect closure, and if the pharyngeal flap, superiorly based, cannot be done, or if the patient has

lost the soft palate, then it becomes necessary to extend our
case into the pharyngeal area and construct a speech appliance, or speech bulb, as it is sometimes called. We refer
to it always as an obturator. The base of the speech appliance must not interfere with swallowing or tongue movements. The eustachian tubes must be free from any impinge-
ment, but the appliance must show an impression of the
posterior and lateral walls of the pharynx. The patient must
be able to effect closure. A check is made by having him
puff out his cheeks or blow up a balloon. Adjustments usually
have to be made. Any irritating areas must be relieved.
Patients may not be able to breathe through the nose while
lying down; then we must relieve the lateral areas of the
speech appliance. Production of mucous may be a factor here.
The anterior area of the appliance must be relieved. It usually
takes about five or six adjustments to correct all these difficulties. When the case is completed to our satisfaction, the
patient is sent back to the speech therapist to receive more
instructions and therapy.

DOCTOR HAWTHORNE: We are going to speak about cases
ranging from birth to the final stage of the primary dentition,
which you think of in terms of three, three, and three; that
is the magic number in dentistry. The final dentition is
usually complete in the child by the age of three. They
keep it for three years and then the six-year molars come
in so this is the next "three." And then, at age nine, the
cuspids and bicuspids start to move around in the jaw and
this is another phase in terms of our treatment. So, outlining it, let us say birth to age three; age three to age six;
and then from six to nine. This is not of too much interest
to the speech people other than the fact that it is an orthodontic phase. Finally we will go into the teenagers and
then the adult phase.

The complete cleft of the lip and the ridge, and the hard
and soft palate, is intercepted as soon after birth as possible,
and before the plastic surgeon closes the lip. The reason
for this is that the plastic surgeon, upon closing the lip,

puts on an awful lot of pressure. When the lip is closed over the alveolar ridge it is like an elastic band going across, and the ridges will close and effect a very marked cross-bite on the side of the cleft. What will happen after the lip is closed? This will come in to cross-bite or be lingual to the mandible in the future with the eruption of the primary teeth.

The next stage is for the dentist to go to the infant ward and take an impression. An impression on these babies is very difficult and there are a number of hazards that we will possibly run into. The number of people necessary to do this is three. Our belief at Children's Hospital is not to anesthetize the child. Many cleft palate centers anesthetize the child and use five people and this is, I think, a waste of paramedical personnel. It is also much more difficult because I want to have the child crying, screaming at the top of its lungs, when I take the impression. Surprisingly enough, I can get some good posterior anatomy and I can have the tongue move this impression material around so that when I make my silastic appliance I do not impinge upon the structures that would possibly cause difficulty in respiration.

The appliance is then formed on a model. The appliance is made out of silastic #382, which is a medical silastic made by Dow-Corning. This silastic is used to make prosthetic appliances throughout the human body. We started doing this in 1964, after extensive research, and the material is tissuphile. It does not present any problems as far as causing ulceration or any harm on the soft tisues in the mouth of the child. The vomerine stalk is sometimes ulcerated because the membrane over it is not as tough as the membranes in the mouth. However, this material will not cause any trouble. The mother can take care of it. She washes it three times a day or whenever she is done feeding the child. It does not cause a fungus growth and the only problem that we have found with it is that it will stain from the baby's formula.

The appliance is placed in the baby's mouth before he goes in for surgery on the lip. As I say, the orbicularis oris muscle will just close that arch right over. We have gotten some dramatic results doing this, creating the growth of bone, and we do not know where the bone comes from. But we have actually found that the maxillary segments tend to grow around this. Maybe it works on the principle that for every action there is an equal and opposite reaction, and this is an irritating factor in some respects; it probably irritates the bone so that the bone grows around it. However, some of our very well versed colleagues do not answer this. Also, we contour this appliance so that there is movement for the tongue and it also acts as a feeding appliance. We tell the mother it is a feeding appliance and we therefore do not have to give her any long explanation. With the appliance, after the lip has been closed, the alveolar ridges start to approximate around the appliance. After the primary dentition start to develop, we like to keep this appliance in the mouth until the palate is closed. Or, even better, but again there is a time and a social factor, if we could wait until the first primary molars erupt the cusps will lock into the molars and will prevent these ridges from collapsing. So it is a timing factor, also. The timing on this is that the lip is closed usually within the first couple of weeks and then the hard and soft palates are closed at approximately fourteen to sixteen months.

Another thing that I want to bring up is the fact that when the palate is closed, we make it very, very rough on Doctor McEvitt because by the child's using this appliance, the doctor no longer has a little gap of maybe four or five millimeters to close. Now his gaps are as big as a centimeter to a centimeter and one-half, and he now has to go into what is called a two-stage operation. He does not like it in that respect, but in the other respect, we have eliminated a lot of dental problems in the future.

So we have achieved the one thing that we want—we have gotten our forward growth of the maxillary segments. They are approximated and butted together. We have also eliminated what was supposedly the vogue a few years ago, and that is that everybody was doing bone grafts; they picked up a book and read about it and they did a bone graft. And this is more surgical trauma to the child. We have found that it is not necessary in many of these cases. The alveolar ridges come together and they will hold in that position. A bone graft is not necessary, other than possibly for a cosmetic purpose of supporting the lip. Surgical trauma is 'one thing we try to get away from.

Now we get to the orthodontic trauma. Without the appliance in place, you will get on the side of the cleft a cross-bite, as we call it, or a lingual locking of the upper teeth in the lower, which is not in the normal dentition. So then we have to start the orthodontic treatment. The orthodontic phase is handled in two ways and is based upon several things. The people in the speech department would rather have us make a fixed appliance. However, if we have a fistula in the area of the cleft, sometimes we will use a re-movable appliance which acts as a plate to cover the fistula and will aid the speech people in helping the child to develop his speech. So we make the type of appliance called a jack-screw. When you hear about a jackscrew, it is a spring-loaded screw, and it is cranked out every so many days. We will let some parents do it, others we have to do ourselves. Some of our parents have difficulty with this. The fistula is covered so that the segment is being moved by tightening the jack-screw and moving the segment without opening the fistula. When the segment is out, we can leave the appliance in the mouth just by filling it in with acrylic.

We do not move teeth. We are not moving teeth yet, we are moving bone—we are moving the maxillary segment. In terms of orthodontics, this is not a pure orthodontic pro-cedure. We have actually moved this whole maxillary seg-ment. And then if we do not get the children at that phase, we get into where it is a complicated mixed dentition with very bad malaligning of teeth, with a need for more compre-hensive orthodontic treatment. These children are usually des-tined to be treated up to age fourteen or fifteen, depending on when treatment is started. As a sidelight which we will bring up in the future, children with clefts have a problem of a high incidence of caries, and the reason for this is that the natural mechanisms in the mouth, i.e. the cheek, the tongue and the lip, act as a self-cleansing mechanism. When there is malaligned dentition, nature's way of taking care of this when you do not have a toothbrush is not as good. So this is one of the reasons for caries. The development of the toothbrush, due to all the other problems the child has, brakes the tooth much more easily to decay in the mouth.

Now we get to the more complicated clefts, and I say more complicated from my viewpoint, because we still have a lot of problems with the bilateral clefts. The worst cleft in the mouth is a bilateral complete cleft of the lip and palate. The lip closure on these children is done in a two-stage operation. They do not close the lip in one stage. However, if Doctor Hawthorne can get in and get the appliance in the mouth before any lip closure is done, we can eliminate a lot of these problems. Again, take note of the fact that with these appliances, we pay attention to the alignment as far as the alveolar ridge goes. And we also contour it so that the tongue does have its free way to move and we are not creating problems for the speech people in the future.

There is also a bilateral cleft where the alveolar ridges are in alignment. We do have the interlocking of the cusps in the proper position in the primary molars. However, there may be some difficulty anteriorly in the future. This is based on growth; some of the surgeons are cutting the vomer and trying to push it back. However, if they cut the growth center in the vomer, the result is the dish-face appearance. In other words, we just eliminate or retard the growth in the middle section of the face. So, cutting the vomer is not a good surgical procedure. It has not proven to be the ideal thing.

There is also a bilateral cleft that is necessarily bone grafted. Bone grafting is not the vogue, but we do it. Bone grafting started approximately twenty years ago, using the crest of the ilium and iliac cartilage. Since that time we have found that this is not the best donor site, so now the rib is used. At first, the rib was taken out *in toto* and the periosteum left in, and then the rib segments were lifted to approximate back. However, in a female, this can create problems as far as her growth goes. So now we have gotten a little more sophisticated and just the top shelf of the rib is taken off. And it is taken off right inside the chest cavity, leaving the bottom half of the rib so there is no malformation in the development of the chest. The piece of rib is taken right out of the chest and is cut in half in the chest, with the bottom half left in. Then the chest cavity is sewn up and we go to the mouth. The child is anesthetized and is on the operating table. In bone grafting, the next step is to make a water-tight, air-sealed pocket. Doctor McEvitt now goes in and makes a pocket to receive the bone first, and dismisses the child. After two or three months, the child returns to have the bone taken out of the chest and put into the pocket. Surprisingly enough, I have seen from bone grafting using a piece of rib, that tooth buds do migrate into this segment. In other words, this bone changes its morphology and becomes alveolar bone. And tooth buds do grow into this area. Then it is closed. The silastic appliance now has a new function; it is keeping the maxillary segments from impinging on this bone graft, allowing the bone graft to take hold and to develop in a normal way.

Orthodontic problems now begin to arise because this child was not born during the right time; he or she did not have the privilege of being treated the other way, so now you find in the bilateral cleft that the premaxilla, rather than being protruded, is retruded; the child does not even have any function of the lower anteriors. Just as a sidelight, these are called "mammalons." The edges of the teeth wear off where the teeth come together. In other words, nature intended these to wear off from biting end to end. However, there is no function anteriorly. So this gets into the complicated orthodontic phase. This will have to be expanded on both sides, making it more complicated, and some type of consideration must be made as to what to do to the premaxilla. We do not routinely remove these if we can help it. In some cases we have to.

In doing our work-ups, as Doctor Sproule said, the most important thing is to get good, adequate records. You do not do a five-minute diagnosis and five years of work. We have developed a way of intercepting these children and making what we call a pretty complete study of x-rays on every child that comes to the Cleft Palate Center; this is done within one hour. So, we can see twelve children in one hour and get a fairly decent start of x-rays by taking three to five x-rays. When you go back to your cleft palate groups, you may find that the group does not have any x-ray diagnosis because they figure it takes a lot of time. But this is a short, sweet, quick way of doing it, and will answer a lot of questions. We can take upper and lower occlusals and the kids love it. You take a picture of their chin and they are not frightened. When you start putting stuff, and your fingers, in their mouth and you have them biting on things, the younger ones all think I am a Hitler when they start screaming, but I can get these done easily. I say, "I take a picture of your nose, I take a picture of your chin, then of your ear." Actually, what I'm doing is taking an x-ray from way behind the ramus of the manible, going to the opposite side, and getting the dentition of the upper and lower to see both the primary and the developing permanent dentition. The child is instructed to bite on a cotton roll; we put a piece of tape over his nose, and with little girls, sometimes we catch their hair in the tape, but that is part of the fun of working on it.

Our prosthetic treatment gets very involved and it is not something that you can do just by hanging a nice little fancy appliance on and expect it to work by reaching out here. Again, we have that principle of the lever. And the lever is the biggest problem in any mouth. For anybody who has any type of dental appliance in their mouth, it is the torquing and the lever forces in the mouth that ruin the teeth and can also ruin the bone and everything else. So we have to consider this especially with the cleft.

Speech people seem most interested in the orthodontic phase. They say, "How long is sweetie-pie going to have the appliance in her mouth, because we are not getting anywhere with her speech?" We try to explain that all they need the teeth for is something to anchor the appliance on; then, that bone moves out nicely. The appliance that I like to use—and it is a silly little appliance; it does not look like much— is called a Porter-W. It gives some of the best moving force that I have found. It is a fixed appliance. I have this appliance in a child who is two and a half years old. This child can not take it out. When we get to the older children, if they get their popsicle sticks, all-day suckers, and such, they pull them out. What we do is hang a three-barb spike here and when anything touches it it puts a hole in it and they stop playing with it.

The Porter-W is put lingually against the teeth. However, the moving force can be directed two ways. It can move a maxillary segment laterally, or it can move individual dental units. And it is a fixed appliance; it is not in the way.

The other problem that we brought up before was the fact that many of these cases have to be intercepted orthodontically, and this is *interceptive orthodontics*. I am not a licensed orthodontist as such, but interceptive orthodontics can be done very adequately by a dentist who cares about doing this, and the results are as you have seen in the past and as you will see in the future. But many times the toothbrush is hanging in the bathroom, and the candy is in the kitchen, and it is a question of which comes first. You never get to the toothbrush, and what you get is rampant decay! All the teeth are decayed, and some cannot be saved. So, with the decay factor, we have to remove teeth and impinge on the speech factor, but these are things that you will find.

Again, orthodontically, here is a case, and it really looks tough. There is lingual lacking in the central, cuspids are locked, and so on. However, with the cooperation of the patient, in using appliances, and with the cooperation of the speech instructor, if there is a speech problem, we go to work,

making our work-up, making our diagnosis, deciding what type
of appliance we are going to use and deciding which type of
patient we have. This is just the case of one year. Orthodontics many times takes two, three, four, or five years if we
get them in the interceptive phase. This is probably being
used around dental circles now because everybody is orthodontic conscious. Ten years ago a kid would not wear braces.
Today it is a social status symbol to have braces. It hurts
children to have their braces off. So if you tell them that they
are going to look like the kids in Bloomfield because they have
braces—man, they will wear them!

By the girl's wearing the appliance, and by our again working in the upper and the lower, having frequent visits, and
adjusting these appliances, we are moving these teeth around.
I have a little locking here in the lateral with the lower cuspid,
and I have one of those wires that you do not like interfering
with the tongue; but, look what we have got—one year. We
did have a speech problem for a year that was possibly being
bothered by orthodontic appliances, but in one year we have
got this all whipped around so that this young lady has a nice,
acceptable dentition. Again, if you notice, the twelve-year molars are not in but the cuspids are, so since this child is approximately eleven or twelve, we did not wait. We did not
procrastinate. We have all the teeth aligned very nicely.

Then we get these; and these are the bad ones where we
cannot really justify taking this out and we cannot justify
saving it. So these malformed teeth that you see in the area
of the premaxilla, in the area of the cleft, because of the self-
cleansing mechanisms in the mouth, decay very rapidly and
many times they will abcess. Thus we have to go into more
comprehensive orthodontics so this is not the one-year deal,
this is more like the two-, three-, or four-year deal. These are
good anterior teeth and all we have to do is just straighten
these around and we are going to use them.

Now, here is a case of a protruding premaxilla. You can
see that the incisal edges of the central incisors are below the
gingiva on the lower and these teeth are of no value; so we

remove them and put in an appliance. This is one of the parts of our work-up where we have to decide what we are going to do. Are we going to perform surgery on this or are we going to keep it? With many cases, as you see with this child, they are past the age where we would try to save it. So this is a condition for removal. You should not treat a temporary appliance as being only temporary. These are transitional appliances which carry the child for from, sometimes, eight to ten years. They carry him through the transitional phase of the development of the arches. Also, the appliances which are going to be made on these cases where the premaxilla has been surgerized allow for the eruption of the other permanent teeth. We can change it around and adjust it now and then until we get to the point where we are going to make our final appliance. So this so-called "temporary" actually is a transitional.

Now we are into the young adult and the adult phase. This is where it takes a lot of treatment planning and diagnosis. Here is a case where we tried to do the best treatment and then work our way down to what ends up being a denture. However, in dentistry, fixed bridge work is best, because this is in the mouth, it doesn't come out, it is attached to the teeth, and this is like your natural teeth. All you have to do is remember they are NOT natural teeth, and anything that is not natural that is put in the mouth requires at least twice as much care as something that is natural. So we instruct our patients by saying, "You have to brush this six times a day rather than three times a day." And they will brush it three times a day, then. So again it is a case of patient education, making them realize the importance of our instructions. I even have a very difficult time in the hospital making trained nurses realize how important those little silastic appliances are. So now, when I put an appliance in a baby, I tell them that appliance represents five thousand dollars. If they lose that, they're throwing five thousand dollars out the window, because if the appliance is lost and we do not do the treatment, it is going to be five thousand dollars by the time that child is twenty-one years old. So all this stuff is very important.

It is not just dentistry; it is not just a dental unit; it is very important, and a cleft palate probably has three times as much value placed on it dentally as a normal mouth.

This is a case of an undeveloped incisor, and as we diagnosed this case, we figured that orthodontic work had already been done. How are we going to treat it? Fixed bridge work was the treatment of choice after making diagnostic models and taking good, adequate radiographs to make sure that the abutments that we are going to put our fixed appliance on are strong—that we are not going to put something on today, and five years from now it will be a failure. So all these things have to be brought into consideration and it is a case, also, of how far do we go. In other words, when you put a bridge on, you do not just cover the bad teeth, but you must figure that you have to get enough retention. So how far around the arch are you going to go? We try to get over to the eyetooth. It is the longest root in the mouth; it is the best anchor tooth in the mouth. So if we take the eyetooth and hook onto it, fine; otherwise, we may go back to the first bicuspid which has two nice roots on it. When these cases are being treated orthodontically, it creates a problem because everything has to be done very rapidly, and we have to make our temporary appliances to hold the orthodontic phase, or else everything else collapses in the meantime. In this case we went from the eyetooth all the way around to an upper molar with three roots, because the leverage on this thing is going to be really something. This is the fixed bridge. Many people call a removable partial a removable bridge. There is terminology that has to be straightened out here. This is a fixed bridge; it is fixed on the teeth and it is there; that is it. This is that same girl, and this is her bridge in her mouth. As far as color goes, it is hard to take slides and to show a blending of color. You can see in the relaxed position that she does have an opening anteriorly.

This is a very interesting case, and I will regress for a minute. We have these models up here, and I have placed them over to one side in a sequence of three. There is a great big hole in the palate. This girl was eighteen when this was taken; this is a large, U-shaped cleft of the palate. These large, U-shaped clefts are not easy to close surgically. So skin grafting is sometimes done. In this case, this young lady had a piece of skin cut off her belly, sewn on to her arm, got circulation in it on her arm, and it was grafted from her arm to the back of her palate. Take a piece of the belly tissue; sew it to the posterior palate; get circulation; cut it off the arm; sew it on the anterior palate; and then what happened? The operation did not take; it got a little infection in it. So they did not completely close the palate, and there is a great big fistula in there.

Another problem with some of these skin grafts is that when a permanent appliance is made, these people have to be given instructions regarding weight control. Because if they gain weight, this still has a lot of adipose tissue in it and this will gain weight and displace the appliance. So, this is another one of our problems. Look, her dentition is almost ideal.

There is surgical orthodontics being done and you end up with nice blue teeth because with surgical orthodontics you get the teeth in position, but they are all dead. So we have to make compensations. Surgical orthodontics is actually cutting the bone and then putting the teeth in position, putting bone chips up there, and you get a beautiful dentition as far as occlusion goes, but nice blue teeth.

As far as occlusion goes, the word occlusion is the matching of the upper and the lower teeth, in the dental sense, and we have keys to occlusion. Many physicians look at patients but they look right past their teeth. All of you look into their mouths at some time or another, so something that all of you can do, and this might help a child, you might be able to intercept a problem that is getting bad. There is a *key* to occlusion. And the *key* to occlusion is the groove on the lower molar and the point mesial or anterior on the upper molar. So, if you look at that, and that point on the upper molar is matching into that groove on the lower molar, you have a good bite. In cases where you have buck teeth, many times the back point on the upper molar will be in the groove of the lower molar. And, when you have an overgrowth of the mandible, many times the point on the upper molar will be between the lower first and second molar. So, one of the keys to occlusion is whether the mesial point matches into this groove. You can tell when a child is seven years old because this is when the molars come in and they go into occlusion. So when we look at occlusion, this is what we look for.

The second thing we look for is that the upper cuspid, the incisal edge on the mesial, is on the distal mesial edge of the lower cuspid, or about half way. The key to occlusion is the first molars. And, again, you can see on this slide, we have some missing teeth, and still we have the key to occlusion. The mesial buccal point of the upper first molar is in the buccal groove of the lower first molar, if you want to know the terminology.

You will see a palatal prosthetic appliance used here not for a dental factor as much as for a speech factor. We did this for you people, and the results we have in models and we have in excellent x-rays that were taken. The x-ray diagnosis on the speech bulb or obturator is done by spraying the posterior palate with barium and covering the bulb with either tin foil or spraying it with barium, and then doing a cinefluoroscopy and radiographs for permanent records. We can then tell whether these bulbs are functioning. They are not just put there for the beauty of it or because some textbooks say to put it on.

The first thing that is done is to find some way to hang this conglomeration of an appliance. We use precision attachments, and the best way to install the appliance is to cover the tooth with a crown. Give that tooth all the adequate protection and all the design for retention. Then it is not as the case of Aunt Minnie who had a partial and lost all her teeth with the partial, because when she had a partial put in her mouth, that was all that was done and her own teeth were not considered at all; Aunt Minnie did not consider the teeth either, so they got decayed and they left the partial, so that the partial was there without the teeth to hang on. So we make precision attachments. These are the attachments. It is a tongue-in-groove; a very, very unique way of doing something, because you have your female attachment like this, and the male attachment. This does not have that much space in it, but this will show you that this is our crown here with the attachment in it, and this is our appliance out here and this fits in. You have to remember that when we do these attachments we do not do one, we do at least two, so everything has got to be parallel. In other words, this groove here has to be parallel to this groove here, and also in doing this, we are not working with something on a bench, we are working with teeth in a human arch that we cannot just sit down and bang and pound and make it fit. So we have to do all this stuff and it takes a lot of time. This gets to be very time consuming and very expensive; however, the results are just beautiful.

Also, here is our appliance and here is our tongue-in-groove. This is a very good picture; you can see our attachments going in here. Why did we do this? Why did we go to this trouble? This is not the end of it, this is just covering that soft belly tissue which is underlying in here, and now Doctor Sproule is going to put a big, long tail on it here. So if you have got this much leverage back here and you have your fulcrum here, you have a darn good means of reciprocation anterior to your fulcrum. This is why we get involved and why we do not treat this in any routine fashion. This gets to be extremely expensive. And this is expensive in another respect. It is gold, but the expense, the initial expense of using a gold partial, is superceded by the fact that gold is like buying a car with nothing on it and then you put all the attachments on it as you go along. The other cases that are less expensive, using the silver-type metal, are electrically welded, and once they are welded, the metallurgy is such that you cannot add on to it.

One other problem is that with some socioeconomic groups I have had nightmares because the pawn shops can use these. If they don't have any money, they might take this to the pawn shop, so we have to stress that this is of value without telling them that it has a monetary value because they may go pawn the denture.

This is looking at the palatal portion in the area of the fistula. Now, again, gold is tissuphile. It is a noble metal; it is the metal of choice against tissue. Actually, the tissue sings when it has gold next to it. The fistula in the girl's mouth, since this appliance has been put there, has actually closed. We do not know why. Doctor Sproule and I sit and look at the models each time she comes in, and this fistula is actually closing up now. Radiographically, we cannot tell whether bone is growing in there or whether it is just soft tissue. The fact is that the fistula is closing. As you can see, this is not polished and there is some irritation. Again, for each action, there is an equal and opposite reaction. So we irritate this tissue a little bit, and this is probably the same thing with our silastic appliances and we cannot prove why we get this, though I think it is the irritation and this is the tissue fighting back. So this is the appliance in the mouth and Susan, again, has been cautioned about gaining weight. I will now let Doctor Sproule take over.

DR. SPROULE: The first step in constructing an obturator is to attach a piece of lead to the appliance and shape it over any soft tissue and into about the center part of the pharyngeal area and put a retentive area across the top. This time we use a compound, a simple compound made of resin and wax material that softens at about the temperature of about 120° and becomes hard at body temperature. This is placed in the patient's mouth in a soft state. The patient is instructed to swallow. We have movements of the head forward, backward, and sideways, and then we have them twist the head from side to side. The compound is removed and checked to see if we have an impression of the areas of the pharynx. Also, we have an impression of the posterior wall of the pharynx. That was the final impression of the bulb. In doing it, I imagine that was in and out of the mouth maybe ten to fifteen times before we finally got to the point where we had complete impressions of the walls. Now the patient is sent home with the appliance in compound in the mouth, and is brought back three or four days later to check for irritations both to the pharynx and to the tonsillar pillars because we have to keep it tight around the pillars and still keep them from being irritated. And when we are perfectly satisfied with the shape in compound, making all our adjustments in the compound first, we use a Harken's paste, which is a very, very thin, soft paste, over top of the compound. It is replaced in the patient's mouth. It becomes very smooth and we send it to the laboratory to have the compound replaced with a clear plastic. When the case is finished, the patient returns and it is set in the mouth, and from then on there are slight adjustments, probably, that have to be made, but there are very, very few because of the work that has been done previously in the compound.

The piece of the appliance that comes across is our bulb or speech appliance. If you will notice, this little drip that you see here is due to the barium that was used on the appliance at the time that they took the x-ray so it will show up definitely in the mouth. It is away from the eustachian tube. The tongue has formed the base of the appliance. The lateral walls will not show here but they have been contoured as you see. When this patient would speak or blow there is complete closure and Doctor Falk checked this patient afterward. We found that that patient with this attachment had a complete closure in the pharyngeal area. Food and water that beforehand had been coming back through the nose was completely eliminated. I do not know if she has gone on with her speech training since that time or not.

DOCTOR HAWTHORNE: Going further into prosthetic cases, we are going to bypass the orthodontics and now we are in the phase where we are going to treat the case at the age of seventeen up to twenty. There are many things that are involved in treating these cases at this time. The biggest problem that we have found is the Frankfort mandibular angle. This is the angle of the mandible studied radiographically. Do you know what this is? It is a mode or a means of measurement, measuring sella tursica. This is the main center of measurement going on a plane across to just below the orbit, i.e. running on a plane from the sella tursica across to the floor of the orbit. I did a study when I was in training with the Merrill-Palmer Institute in which we had x-rays that were taken of people in the forty-year-old bracket and we got the people back when they were in the fifty-year-old bracket. After ten years there was still growth in the mandible. So there is always growth.

So, this angle, if it is steep like this—again, here is the sella tursica up here—if this angle is steep we have found that these children have a growth spurt, in especially females, at the age of seventeen or eighteen. So in these cases we have tried to use mainly social pressure because they want to go out and get married. They want to have an appliance in their mouth. Fine! But the appliance is put in the mouth and two years later it is dentally a failure; it still might look good to them, but we have lost all the function of occlusion and everything else because of that growth phase shooting the mandible forward. In these cases we try to put them off, using a transitional appliance or some other means of treatment, until they are approximately twenty because then this growth is down to its minimum, and the appliance will usually hold. On the other hand, it has been found sometimes that an appliance can be made to approximate these teeth. It will lock this and prevent some of this growth. Maybe this happens; we do not know. So I am going to bring that up. I just wanted to show that to you now so you have it in mind.

In treatment, as I have said, a denture is the last choice; the choice is fixed. We went through fixed, and now the next choice is what they call a fixed-removable appliance. We try to keep it as fixed as possible, but for some reason we have to make it removable. So, I am going to show you a natural case. This is an auto accident case where this gal broke all her front teeth out and even lost bone in the area of the maxilla. This is a normal case, this is not a cleft, but I want to show you this and how the principle was applied very nicely a couple of times since then to a cleft palate. Anterior to the second bicuspid, there is only a small amount of ridge tissue. However, because of the ridge tissue and the maxilla, supporting of the lip could not be accomplished by putting in a fixed bridge. A fixed bridge would be a bridge with teeth all the way around it. So instead we make a platinum bar, and the platinum bar is going to be our clothesline, more or less. Here is this ridge. Again, this is the incisive papilla, which is the little lump on the inside of the mouth that hurts when you eat a pizza or a bagel or something. An this is the end of her alveolar ridge, which is posterior to the lower anterior teeth. We had to come out, we had to fill this all out and bring everything anterior to the incisal edges of the lower teeth. So we made crowns. And, again, remember the biggest crown in the mouth is a lever. So, anything that goes—here is our fulcrum—anything that goes here has got to be well compensated-for posterior to it as a reciprocal means of holding this. We used upper molars— they have three roots—so we have three roots on the upper molars, we have two roots on the first bicuspid, we have good holding power, good anchorage. Then this is put in the mouth and an impression is taken. This is formed on a jig. But an impression is again taken of this and we make these out of wax first. We can add, subtract, fill in the lip and give them the function, get plumping out in the lip and so on. And then this appliance slides over. Now, here is the inside of the appliance, and these again are little clamps that go over more than half way around that bar. And as added retention, we have a tongue-in-groove effect, though not quite as fancy as a precision attachment. The reason is that when you start getting eight different units parallel to each other, it is almost impossible to do it. So, we have to change our treatment in some respects. Now here it is in the mouth. And you can see how far foward we had to go. With a bridge, also, you could hang teeth on the bridge but you could not get the alveolar ridge approximation as far as filling the lip out into its position. Here it is filling out in the area of the filtrum. And that is it in the patient's mouth.

Here is a cleft palate patient who was orthodontically treated. We moved the alveolar ridges out, we moved the bone out, and we had the teeth that were there in good position, but if you look at the alveolar ridge, you see this big area. This is a depression and you can see how the depression is here on the lip. This is very good surgery, but if you look at it from a side view, there is a depression in there. And you cannot fill this all up with a bridge. Also, if you put a bridge in, the patient will have difficulty in keeping it clean. The cleanliness factor is important, also, and is another consideration in doing this. So the teeth are good. This is one thing that really makes you hesitant to subject good teeth to dental intervention. Any tooth that is good is better than cutting it and putting a crown on. But you have to make decisions in certain problems like this. And we have to get anchorage.

Let us look at the palate. Here, again, is a depression. And you want those tongues for articulating, and you have a lot of articulative surfaces here that are not as good as normal, smooth contoured palates. Again, in this case, the teeth were good. So, we did not want to go all the way around routinely to the cuspid. We had the opportunity of having a good incisor and two bicuspids and we did not have to extend it as far forward as we did in the other case. We do not need that reciprocity posterior to the fulcrum. We got our occlusion, we have our bar in there, and then we make this nice little prosthetic appliance using the same principle but this time sticking a long tailpiece on it to fill in that palatal depression. Now, it is lying in this palatal depression. And now we have a nice smooth contoured hard palate in the anterior area and a nice articulating surface for the tongue.

This girl had a steep, steep Frankfort mandibular angle, and her jaw practically went right from the tip of her ear down with hardly any angle in the corner of the mandible. So, she has a bilateral crossbite. She has this mixed dentition. As a matter of fact, she is a skinny little thing because she could not even eat right.

The first thing we did, before we approached this, was to fashion a wax rim. We stuck it into the mouth to see how we could bring this lip out because you have to have your lips together to swallow. You also have to be able to bring those lips together. So many times, the tension on this lip tissue is such that you cannot just routinely bring everything out as far as any normal contour. You have to be able to bring it out, so you take the wax, you cut the wax, you get your approximation of how far anteriorly you can bring out the prosthetic appliance. Then we got rid of eleven teeth and left three. So we have two three-rooted molars and one long-rooted cuspid. Everything else was removed. What do we do here? This is a very, very rough problem dentally because we are going to use precision attachments and it is hard enough to get this unit parallel to this unit. But when you have a tripod and to get this unit and this unit and this unit all parallel so that it all slides in on something that is not stable, it is a natural entity, and it is hard to do this—to get them all parallel. Therefore, we make three crowns. Again, because of the design of this appliance, these crowns had no functional anatomy. There is no need to have functional anatomy. But they have something that is much more functional. Not only are these three grooves parallel to each other but also, even though the teeth were not parallel, the crowns are cast and made parallel. The parallelism gives added retention. It has been found in the past with many dental interventions in the cleft palate that there is enough stress on these that you can put an appliance in, and we find it with our transitional appliances, that they will just pop out after a while because they are not being held. So, you cannot approach by undercutting. Undercutting it is just too hard. You try to approach getting every tooth parallel to the other one so they work harmoniously together as anchors. And remember we have to go all the way out to here to consider the palate with our appliance. You have to get as much retention as possible.

This is an articulator. An articulator, as Doctor Sproule says, duplicates the movements of the jaw, and also an articulator relates the maxilla to the condyle. This is the temporomandibular joint relation to the articulator. And an anatomic articulator is the only way you can study many of these cases. You set it up and find out exactly how it is going. You cannot have him just bite into a piece of mush and stick it on a barn door hinge. You have to use something that will give us all the relationships we want. We can get into some very fancy articulators but this is not for this group.

We can see now that surfaces are parallel. We try to get everything as close to giving adequate retention so it just really holds. Again this is a gold case. And I am glad it was a gold case because we learned something. This jaw grew, so we had to eliminate all the acrylic that had the teeth and added on to it again and it did not create any major expense problem. The expense was in the beginning and not in the end.

This is looking at the attachment that we've been talking about. Again, you can see this is about a three millimeter jump from the edge of the alveolar ridge to the incisal edges in the mandibular centrals. The appliance is then put in her mouth. And there it is and those are our teeth. And here, you can see, you get an approximation of how steep this angle is in the mandible. And here it is from the side view. Beautiful! Look at this! You can just lay your stick here. There is hardly any ramus in the mandible.

DOCTOR SPROULE: You will notice that the relationship of the jaws here, the tip of the chin to the nose, is close. Now this is when we started working in the final part of the case. You notice how the upper lip is depressed. First of all, Doctor Hawthorne crowned these teeth. As a matter of fact, in all our work we work a great deal together so that we are both very familiar with each one of them. Teeth were crowned. Impressions were taken. This is a photograph of a transitional that was made when the patient was about eight or nine years of age, which she had worn for a period of ten years. All along the way adjustments had to be made so that she could appear, go to school, speak well, and still be able to masticate her food. Even with a plastic base on the transitional, I used a stainless steel tongue that was fastened, and the speech appliance was formed into the pharyngeal area. This functioned very, very well for the period of time that she had to wear it.

Now we came to the final work. Doctor Hawthorne, as I said before, crowned the teeth. And this is a case where we used nothing but clasps on these teeth. The crowns were formed and adequate retention was made on the forming of the crowns so that the clasps could clasp around these teeth and be strictly firm. The case was made of gold, so that attachments could be made later. There are the crowns in place brought into occlusion. The case was first waxed up. The teeth were set into occlusion and on an articulator, as we have explained before, set into position for the best speech possible and the inside of the palatal area was contoured. I ran into a little difficulty in the contouring of the palate to give sufficient room for the tongue in the sibilant sounds.

This is the case completed. Notice the contour of the palatal area. Shadows will show the contouring of that palatal area. The tongue was attached to the posterior part of the appliance. The impressions were taken for the bulb by means of compound, as we always do, and was worn in compound until we had made all of our adjustments. The adjustments all completed, the case was finished into a clear plastic. And I saw the patient yesterday and she is now working and getting along very, very well. She should have more speech training, however.

That is the inside of the case. You will notice the shape of the bulb in the posterior area. You can see the way that the posterior part of the pharynx has shaped that bulb. Also, the lateral walls shape the lateral areas of the bulb. And reliefs have been made in the area of the eustachian tubes. We have a hearing difficulty. We get infections of the ear and hearing difficulty then is reflected in speech. Therefore, all these factors have to be taken into consideration at the time the bulb is made. There is a good deal of difficulty in getting this gal to smile.

This case was presented to me—a man about forty-five years of age. I was never able to find out exactly whether he had had surgery done and it had been a failure or not, because he just did not remember. He has lost the complete palate. He wore this type of appliance for a number of years. It had absolutely no contour to it and it did not function as a speech appliance. The only thing that it did was to sit up into the palate and give him something to chew with. And he is complaining at this time that people are not able to understand him. This was his big complaint. So it was a speech therapist in Windsor that sent him to Detroit to see if something could be done for him.

In this case, we had the advantage of having five upper teeth. As we said before, we crown these teeth. These particular teeth were not crowned as ordinary teeth would be crowned. They were crowned, the teeth were parallel, but the crowns were cone shaped and we refer to this as a telescope crown because we are going to make our appliance over top of these crowns and use them strictly as a stabilizing agent. The appliance was made, and you will notice that the crowns are all parallel. The teeth were set up first in wax; we tested what articulation we could get. Then we completed the case. Before I put the final plastic on, I added a tail to it. Also, at the time the casting was done, you will notice that across the top of it, I ran a little retentive area along in through here, which I will show the reason for later. The bulb was fashioned in the mouth in the usual way. You can definitely see the impressions of the lateral walls. The tonsillar pillars that were left came in through here.

I added plaster to this little retentive area that I showed

you just previous to this. It came straight through and followed right through to the anterior region. This is an artificial vomer. That was not added until later because I wanted to be sure, definitely, how the speech bulb was working and also check on the resonance that we were having. I found that by placing that artificial vomer in, the resonance of his voice improved tremendously. Since that time, we have made further adjustments on that and each time that we make an adjustment, the speech is improved. That is the case as it stands and you can see that the vomer area has been carried through to the anterior region. Here I have added more compound, trying to effect a better closure and get better resonance and better speech. By the way, he wears a full upper and full lower.

DOCTOR HAWTHORNE: These are little goodies we call anomalies. This child has no tongue. And as we talked about the self-cleansing mechanisms of the tongue, the cheeks and the lips, does he have decay! No self-cleansing! The upper is not bad. You can see how important your tongue is, not only for speech but also for just keeping the teeth clean when you do not use a toothbrush. Here is a little bulb that is the area that is supposed to be the tongue. This is all the floor of the mouth, here. This is probably the sublingual gland in this area. Here again, there is what was supposed to have been a tongue.

These are things that you can take back and say, "Gee, I finally saw one." This is, again, a method of prosthetically treating a case. In this case, the work that was done was in early life when the child was about eleven or twelve. You can see that the difficulty is that the premaxilla has been operated on and lost due to one reason or another. I did not start this case so I do not have some of the information. But now he comes into the office, and he has an overjet of the lower jaw. You can see that thick muscle tissue. But a man does have an advantage since he can grow a mustache and this will hide a lot of errors. I encouraged the patient to start doing this. This case was treated in two phases.

Number one, before we approached the prosthetic treatment, we could take advantage and do some orthodontics. Now, the orthodontics here was accomplished by doing some selective extracting of two bicuspids. If you do not have room to pull everything else back, you can take out two bicuspids and this is called "serial extractions." In a great many cases, they will take out four, and then you pull the other teeth back into the area.

This is the upper palate. And this child was wearing a transitional appliance. But there were very few teeth with which to work. We had to select which ones we were going to keep and which ones we were going to get rid of. So in this case we used the precision-attachment telescope and then anatomically carved crowns with deep rests, as we call them. You can see on this model that now the teeth have been straightened out. Remember, when you bring forward your maxillary segment and you make that lever so great, it is better to find a halfway point. In many cases, when we do have an abundance of alveolar bone and teeth lingual to the lower teeth, we can tip the lower teeth back first and then not have to go out as far with the upper teeth, which is done in this case.

This is, as Doctor Sproule mentioned, a waxing. The waxing is tried in the mouth. The wax can be contoured, the teeth can be repositioned and a lot of adjustments can be made in the wax before it is finally processed, as we call it. This keeps us out of trouble and gives us a lot to work with. You can see we have brought these back and that they were out like this. We got them straight up and down and we get nice alignment which gives us an advantage here. But, pay attention to the fact that he had what they call a "dish face". He was retruded in the maxillary area due to the loss of the premaxilla.

This is what we call a *deep rest* or *lugs*. These give us further retention. Remember we have this fulcrum effect so if you get some pressure on here, we have the clasp ring here to hold it. We have enough pressure in the other area so it does not go down. And it is made out of gold, again, so if there is any need to add on to it, fine. And this is the appliance. What is this up here? Well, what we did was to give him this filtrum that is more cosmetically acceptable. We added on with acrylic to the rim of the denture to give him a filtrum and it is called *pimpling* or *plumping*. It is a cosmetic way of helping this lip. Also, many times it is very tense at first so we have the patient take cocoa butter or some sort of petroleum jelly and massage this to loosen up his lip. Here we are with the appliance in his mouth and you can see that we have orthodontically brought these teeth back.

Another approach is the telescoping of teeth, though many times telescoping is not the only answer. In other words, you put a thimble within a thimble, one being larger than the other. In this case here, we designed a groove in the thimble so that we have a thimble and a groove. Again, the whole thing is based on retention. You put these huge appliances in the oral cavity and you must have retention. There is a lot of movement out here. This young lady is not finished yet because again we found this deep Frankfort mandibular angle of her mandible. She is still growing.

This is what we call a *framework*. A framework is the first step in making these partials and then to this framework you can add or subtract. The framework is a precision casting. It is casted and it fits all of the crowns so that with the framework and with the crowns, the rest can be added or subtracted. You do not have to remake these cases over and over again. We could not, because of this steep angle, get more than an end-to-end bite. We could not get an overbite.

Remember that a Class-I bite is an overbite with the upper anterior teeth biting over the lower anterior teeth. The Class-II bite is the buck-tooth type where there is a large, extreme overbite. For a while, it was thought that that was a very serious problem, but the most serious is the Class-III. That is where the lower teeth bite in front of the upper teeth. So, again, for your terminology, there are three classifications of biting. The Class-III bite is the hardest to treat normally, and then with the cleft, it is also very difficult to treat. You can see that you get this turning down at the corner of the lips and it makes for a real cosmetic problem. You can see we still do not have this. If you would drop a plumb line, you would still touch the chin. And she has grown since.

In treating these, we try to add the teeth or push the teeth out further on the partial. But in some cases, the patient will become subjected to what we call a *resection*. That is, they will take a piece out of the mandible and push the jaw back. And I think that this young lady is going to be destined for one.

This is another one of our anomalies. What does this boy have? Micrognathia. What is micrognathia associated with when you have this bird-face look? Pierre Robin syndrome.

This girl is seventeen. She never developed any permanent teeth. So, orthodontically, the teeth, the permanent molars and the alveolar ridge of bone, everything, has been moved to get an approximation. You have a big hole and you have some very badly decayed teeth. These are primary teeth. And the orthodontic phase is not quite complete. But all that we really want to do is get it out so that this tooth here is over here. You do not need those anterior teeth. She is still moving a little bit. We are going to take advantage of the other teeth and we can also see, again, it is not a case where we are going to do fixed work because we have this big opening in here. So, we have to use a removable appliance, rather than a fixed. That stainless steel crowned tooth was also primary. A stainless steel crown is less of a type of crowning than a gold crown, but in primary teeth it works out very nicely. So now we have these position ridges and we crown the teeth with permanent crowns.

It is a big advantage to try a waxing in the mouth and make the adjustments there rather than making the adjustment on the articulator, thinking that you have something. The crowns are put into occlusion and we have the nice grooves from the precision attachments. We really accomplished something in using a precision attachment, removable partial denture, and being able to build out the lip and give the child contour.

Many times after we do this, we have given Doctor McEvitt a foundation where he can go back and do some cosmetic adjustment if there is not too much scar tissue. The more scar tissue there is, the less successful Doctor McEvitt's treating the lip is because you cannot work on it. And it is very hard to work on. This lip was just as tight as a string on a bull fiddle and so we had to do something as far as trying to get the lip into contour and to give this young lady, who was very small for her age, some cosmetic restoration and function. No function, nothing, only a few anterior teeth treated somewhere else was the treatment of choice. If something is bad, many people just say "Take it and get rid of it." We do not. We try to save every tooth until the last minute and then we will remove them.

Here is a pattern similar to the earlier one. Actually, here is a cuspid, and a bicuspid here, and the bicuspid should be back here. And the same is true here, so that the pattern of eruption is totally disorganized. The treatment is *telescoping;* telescoping being a thimble within a thimble, but keeping it as close to being parallel as possible; a tin can without a tin can, but it does not work in the mouth. This is retentive enough for this case. Also, we used a full palate because in testing out for function as far as speaking was concerned, we found that a full palate gave better anatomy than the palate that had the surgery on it. In the area of the tuberosities, as Doctor Sproule explained in his opening speech, is where we have to sometimes add or subtract for the passage of air. Then just looking in to the mouth here, we could not use a pimple. I would have loved to use a pimple, but when I used a pimple here, because of this tight, tight band of tissue, she just could not bring her lips together. Now that was really going far, and as it was, there was home-care instruction—massage and pull on it to try and get that lip a little looser. Doctor Sproule will take this next case.

DOCTOR SPROULE: This is a patient around the forty-year

age. You can see the position of the upper lip before we started
work. She was much retruded. The teeth, as we have gone
through before, were crowned—crowned for a very definite
reason. To show you our reason, you will notice the collection
of food particles around the edge of these crowns. This patient
has received good instruction on mouth care, but still, if that
was a natural tooth, if those food particles were allowed to
remain in that area, we would have decay in six months, and
loss of teeth and destruction of the appliance. The appliance
was made using thimbles and clasps on the posterior teeth.

After the case was set up and tried in the mouth, and worn
for a short time to get rid of irritations in the anterior area,
the speech bulb was made and set in the mouth. This is the
anterior, or inside, area of the denture with the plumping in
the anterior to bring out the lip as we thought it should be for
aesthetics. This is the case in the mouth. The palatal area is
contoured. You will notice how the tonsillar pillars come in
and form themselves around the speech appliance. This is
important in this area because with a leak through that area,
it is just as bad as if it were in the posterior part of the
pharynx.

DOCTOR HAWTHORNE: I am going to show one quick slide
talking about the importance of this transitional appliance; the
reason being because this is where a lot of work that is put off
should be started. In other words, you don't put something
off because the child is not ready for it due to growth or development. A transitional appliance has many, many uses. And
as we have seen in our whole presentation today we start them
with a transitional even to the point of getting them used to
having something foreign in their mouth. Make them realize
it is a training aid. It has a thousand advantages. It is not
just a transitional as such, but it has a number of different uses.

This boy has a steep Frankfort mandibular angle and is
going to have a lot of growth in that mandible. Why go in
at this time and put in something of a permanent vein and
have it be a failure? It is not good for one's reputation, and
it is not good for the patient as far as their training goes. So

on this transitional, if you will notice in the anterior area, it has all been cut out. This allows for growth and development of the permanent teeth. This allows them to come through, as you can see, without being impinged upon, but at the same time making this boy socially acceptable and giving him the adequate cosmetics he needs so he is able to go out and compete.

Chapter 9

THE ROLE OF THE ORTHODONTIST
IN TREATMENT OF CLEFT
LIP AND PALATE

J. Hilliard Hicks

THE LOGICAL QUESTION that arises in a group like this is why should we be subjected to orthodontic instruction; how will this help us be more effective; why must we learn a new and additional set of terms and the jargon that goes with an additional discipline? For this I have a very good answer. The reason you must do this is that no other groups share such sustained and protracted overlapping of efforts, with the consequences of conflict or cooperation. The speech therapist and the orthodontist see the cleft palate child over the greatest sustained length of time of any of the disciplines. A surgeon is in and out. The prosthodontist is in and out. The orthodontist and the speech therapist inherit these problems for five, six, and seven years. Now these can be five, six, or seven years of pleasant, synergistic effectiveness or they can be six or seven years of bickering, cross-purposes, and misunderstanding; all of which, obviously, will accrue to the detriment of the final result for the child.

The role of the orthodontist in cleft lip and cleft palate therapy is primarily in correction of malocclusion which is required by practically every child who has these defects. In addition, the orthodontist can assist other disciplines concerned in the habilitation and the rehabilitation of the cleft palate child. He can contribute to the assessment of dentofacial growth and development. He can cooperate with the speech therapist for the correction of malocclusion. He can advise the plastic surgeon on the dentofacial growth progress and potential of the patient. In cooperation with the prosthodontist, he can provide orthodontic therapy in conjunction with prosthesis. The orthodontist determines whether growth and development of the jaws and teeth are proceeding normally in the presence of the cleft lip and palate. He constructs attachments for prosthetic appliances and moves teeth into positions favorable for retention, aesthetics, and mastication.

Early orthodontic therapy is required to prevent or correct collapse of the dental arch after the lip is closed surgically. Treatment in the deciduous dentition when the roots show advanced resorption can prove disappointing. Removable appliances should be used where possible in the early mixed dentition or even in the deciduous dentition.

It is impossible to make an orthodontist of anyone in a morning, but if we can teach you what the objectives are, what the limitations are, the names of a few of the critical areas in time of treatment, and reason for treatment, this will help you make a reasonable judgment as to reasons for delay in therapy, stepping up intensity of therapy, and if you speak our language, making requests for changes in types of appliances. Such knowledgeable request is always treated with more respect than one vaguely asking, "Well why don't you do this and that with the thingamajig that was there last month?" Few dentists, indeed, listen or respond to this, but if you convey a semblance of knowledge, the average dentist involved in this type of treatment (and for many of you there will not be a local orthodontist) if he hears five well-chosen words that seem to be part of the jargon, will sit up very straight and take notice because he probably does not know more than seven of these words himself. This makes you doubly effective. You create respect in your own area, but more important, you increase the quality of response in the other co-worker. The only justification for even giving a program of this kind must be the increased welfare of the child-patient who receives the benefits of what little you can take back from here or what little I may offer you.

Both disciplines, the orthodontic specialist and the speech therapist, encounter a mutual problem in occupying not only the same space timewise, but actually the same space physically. The area in which you choose to work is the area in which we sometimes hang rather grotesque and barbaric devices. If you realize that not always are these devices needed right now, if you realize that you can reasonably ask if there is a simpler, better way, a less cumbersome way to do it, you very frequently can influence the orthodontist and you can have your own way. This makes your job more comfortable, more effective, and less frustrating. You should realize that some of the things I am going to tell you are going to seem rather elementary and in the way of a review, but we must be sure that everyone understands where this specialty fits into the general scheme of things. So I am going to review with you, and I hope those who know all about this will be just a little patient.

First, I will discuss the various specialties in dentistry so that you are sure that you know what an orthodontist really is because names of all of these specialties end up with an -ontist. Hence, it can be a little confusing. First of all you have the family dentist, the general practitioner, who has rather unrestricted, broad, ill-defined areas of responsibility, but he also is the man to whom in rural areas you must frequently turn for assistance. This is particularly true if you do not have a palate center available. A good capable family dentist who takes a little interest in a cleft palate child and will work with you and follow your suggestions can frequently be the difference between success and failure in the management of the early stages of this child's dental problems. I am sure that the family dentist is willing to accept your suggestions.

The general-practice dentist is actually anxious to find a

way to supplement his rather meager knowledge of the cleft palate child because he does not usually see any more of these youngsters than you do and most dentists are afraid of doing the wrong thing; consequently, they do nothing and this is the worst possible approach to the problem. If you will augment the family dentist's little knowledge with some reasonable suggestions, in a great many instances, you will at least arouse enough interest so that he will seek additional help. Many of these programs in the outer areas can be very well handled locally after having a primary visit and comprehensive analysis made by a center or by a well-qualified specialist.

In other words, if you have the treatment responsibility of a youngster, you may find that no one in the area is willing to accept the masterminding of the dental problem. Then, your suggestion should be to the parent, and with the consent of the dentist, to go to a cleft palate center or to a well-qualified individual orthodontist. Here you should have a treatment plan outlined, then bring it back where it will bolster the confidence of your family dentist to the point where he will look at paragraph three, line two, where it says on November sixth I am to remove four permanent teeth and he will do it. This he would never dare do on his own without some such authorization, or without somebody else whom he feels is better qualified to take the blame, in case there is serious risk in faulty judgment. Therefore, do not hesitate to seek out help from a local dentist, but plant the seed, at least an inkling of the fact, that as far as you are concerned, unless he has some particular and peculiar knowledge apart from that of the average, minimally trained dentist, would it not be a good idea if these parents could just take this child down to some palate center, have a treatment plan made, come back home, have this plan followed, then if the youngster goes off the main road into the ditch again, you can always go back and get another reassessment?

There is no absolute way that you can look at a youngster and predict what this child will need all through the developmental period, yet this is what I am supposed to do in outlining or making an orthodontic determination of the future growth hazards in this child.

The average dentist does not see enough of these children to ever have a chance to make all of the mistakes necessary to find out what can or will go wrong, and thus to do the next one right. There are just not enough children to go around to let you do something a little wrong each time and finally come up with the right answer. And there is not enough time. There is only one period in this child's development when just a little bit of treatment can be the most effective. If you take eight to ten years of the child's life and blow it on improper treatment, you never have another chance to come back and treat that child as an eight-year-old child when the treatment should have been right. You must be right the first time. And yet when they bring this infant with the palate to the orthodontist, they give you the little acorn and they say, "Now here is the little acorn; you look at that acorn and tell me how tall will this oak be five years from now; how wide will this oak be twelve years from now; which way will the branches lean?" This is what you are expected to do. Well, you cannot be this good. Nobody could be this good. But you are obligated to have a plan. You must start somewhere. So, you have a plan with the idea of revising it when proven wrong as you go down the path toward eventual maturation, the eventual morphology. No one knows what the genetic background of this infant is; yet you must decide, "Should we do a bone graft now; should we expand the palate with a silastic plate; should we section the mandible?" You cannot expect to be infallible; you cannot expect anyone else to be infallible. But, you certainly can avoid making disastrous mistakes by seeking competent help from those who, unfortunately, over the years have made an awful lot of mistakes but are now determined not to make the same ones over again.

After the family dentist, the first specialist that you contact would be a pedodontist. Now what is a pedodontist? A pedodontist is a dentist who has graduate training in management of the problems of preadolescent dentistry. They usually restrict their practice to, up to and including, the fourteenth year. This varies in certain areas. They are particularly adept in handling the children that are inclined to be management problems—the psychologically disturbed child, the resentful child—but more important than this, they usually have, with their graduate training, enough authority and enough stature to deal with the problem parent who, as a rule, is the reason for the problem child. And the pedodontist is naturally available only in rather large areas because it simply takes a community of at least eight thousand people to have enough interested parents who think that their children require more than just minimal dental service.

After the pedodontists, we have a group called the exodontists. These are dentists who have had graduate training in the surgical aspects within the mouth—the removal of teeth, the elimination of cysts, and surgery in the mouth and jaws. Most of their practice is confined to the removal of teeth. They usually have extensive additional training in the use of general anesthesia, and in many of your youngsters general anesthesia is the only way in which a child with massive dental problems can be successfully managed. So you may have reason to seek the services of an exodontist. Exodontists with exceptionally advanced training and from certain well-qualified and specified schools are also oral surgeons, and the oral surgeon does more extensive work, of course, than the exodontist. Oral surgeons will repair palates, repair lips, and treat neoplasms, growths, tumors, and so forth. These men are usually in large teaching institutions, university hospitals, and not readily available for routine care.

We also have specialists who call themselves periodontists. The periodontist is a dentist who has, by additional training, and unfortunately, sometimes merely by courtesy, set himself up as being particularly qualified to deal with diseases of the soft tissue—the supporting tissue of the teeth. This would be the man who treats a disease which we loosely call gingivitis or pyorrhea and who frequently adjusts the bite to relieve a traumatic occlusion and who tries to delay the ravages and the deterioration that accrue to anyone's bone and tissue support over a period of time. Primarily, he is the man who packs pockets, who tries to fix or immobilize loose teeth so that they can become functional and just delay the eventual loss. The periodontist requires a certain resigned fatalism, since they realize that all they can do is fight delaying actions. This isn't quite true in very young patients, but as a rule, they simply fight a delaying action until such time as you have to see the next group of specialists, which is the prosthodontists.

The prosthodontist is a dentist who is specialized and trained in the production, the fitting, and the maintenance of replacement prostheses and missing parts. This is a restricted field very much in its own right since very little in the way of cleft palate prosthodontia is taught in any school, including even graduate schools. Most of these men have had to learn by a process of cut and fit, trial and error. Unfortunately, in the country there have developed strong personalities in this field who have gathered about them dedicated disciples; so we have very divergent philosophies in small pockets all over the United States, which produces a bit of a hazard. A youngster is adequately handled here, for instance, with a certain philosophy, but since we are dealing with a mobile group of people (they work for automobile plants) they get shifted, they change jobs and may suddenly move to California and the man in California throws up his hands in horror and says, "This must have been done somewhere up in the Arctic Circle; I have never seen anything like this." And by the same token, we feel that way about what they do in southern California. These pockets of emotionally active disciples permeate this field extensively, and I guess there is nothing you can do about it except build up a little bit of a nonaggression pact between the various areas in this field and do the best you can. Fortunately, for the child, regardless of which way they go at this stage of treatment, when they require prosthodontic help, you do not make an irrevocable decision because when it comes to a prosthesis, if you do not like the way this one was made, it is something you can discard and do it the other way. At least, there has not been any irrevocable damage. This is not true in the surgical field; this is not true in the orthodontic field, but fortunately, no matter which way you guess in the prosthetic field, you cannot be completely disastrous to the child.

Aside from the prosthodontist, we have a great many quasispecialists. We have, for instance, a group of endodontists. The endodontist is the man who specializes in the maintenance of nonvital or so-called "dead" teeth. If a tooth is fractured, suffers a blow, or if through caries the blood supply is exposed or the tooth abscesses, these are the men who go in there with very precise little files, remove the old blood vessels, remove the putrescent tissue, and do a "root canal," filling and sealing it off, and surgically remove the tip of the tooth. You now have a functional tooth; a nonvital, dead tooth; no blood supply. It actually is a foreign body, except that it is tolerated and accepted and this is a very important adjunct to our work and also the work of the prosthodontist because, unfortunately, almost all of the children with cleft palate and harelip problems have less than average caries resistance. Almost all of them have very bad mouths, principally because the local dentist is afraid to tackle them, and secondly, because the parents are possibly discouraged and try to avoid anything connected with the child's mouth and think that if they do not look in there, maybe it will go away. Consequently, by the time we get them, the most important teeth in this youngster's mouth may already be abscessed; they may be nonsalvageable by any other means except in the hands of an endodonist who can preserve this tooth and give us a fixed and stable anchorage point to go ahead and do more extensive work later.

These are essentially the dental specialties that you will be concerned with. The others, some of them, are pretty far out and will certainly not come into any form of mutual play with your problems.

I have left the orthodontist till last. I assume that most of you know what an orthodontist is. An orthodontist is a man who has been trained to study the growth and development of the teeth, the jaws, and their associated structures, and to correct any deviations or malpositions, in these areas. There are many different types of orthodontic treatment. To understand what an orthodontist is trying to do, you must have some appreciation of what the normal is. You must realize, if you forget everything else I tell you, and remember this, that a cleft palate malocclusion is not an entity in itself. A cleft palate malocclusion is a malocclusion that is superimposed on top of any other anomaly that would accrue to any noncleft child. In other words, a youngster can have an overdeveloped mandible and have a cleft palate, in addition. He can have a micrognathia—a diminutive lower jaw—and in addition, a cleft palate. He may have individual variations in the alignment of teeth and superimposed on this, a cleft palate. He can have congenitally missing teeth; we have any number of children with twelve and fourteen permanent teeth missing— no tooth buds—and superimposed on this is a cleft palate. The cleft palate as such is not a specific type of malocclusion; it is simply an additional deformity imposed on some other type of anomaly or imposed on what would otherwise be a developmentally normal one.

Now, perhaps Doctor Hawthorne told you a little bit about the normal occlusion. Normal occlusion is an occlusion in which the upper arch is essentially outside the lower arch wherein each tooth interdigitates the way gears would interdigitate— where you have each tooth standing vertically in a normal axial position and where the functional movement of the mandible is equal forward, back, right, left. A lot of things happen to prevent this from accruing. While this is normal and what you are entitled to, this is something you very rarely get, and I am not talking only about the cleft palate child. I am talking about any of us. If one side of the maxilla collapses and goes inside the mandible, this can be from posture, it can be from a cleft. You have an anomaly called a cross-bite. The

reason it is a crossbite is that the position of the teeth is reversed. Instead of the upper teeth being on the outside of
the lowers all the way around one side, or even both sides,
the upper arch is inside the lower arch. This is not a very
scientific term, but it is the most common of all the occlusal
problems in a cleft palate child. It is scientifically called a
maxillary collapse, a maxillary contraction, or an inner-canine
growth failure, but it is just, in the lingo, a crossbite.

A normal occlusion is very desirable but it is seldom attainable in most cleft palate youngsters. Rather you try to
achieve a reasonable goal of cosmetic acceptance and functional adequacy, but it will not be normal occlusion in the
sense that we use it with a noncleft child. For this reason,
in the average cleft palate, we have deficiency in the dimension of the upper arch to the point where it cannot possibly
be expanded to go beyond the dimensions of the mandible.
In addition, usually, there are three, four, maybe five tooth
buds destroyed in the line of the cleft or at the time of the
surgery. This is the basic reason why most of the cleft palate
children seem to have a pugnacious—a prognathic—lower jaw;
the little bulldog appearance which is really an optical illusion.
In most of these cases, the mandible is absolutely normal. But
the deficient maxilla gives the appearance of an overgrown
mandible. Since we cannot replace the missing bone, since
we cannot dream up tooth buds that have been lost, we must
approach this by actually creating a commensurate defect in
the lower jaw, which means we frequently remove teeth that
are permanent from the lower arch so that this lower arch
can be contracted down to the point where it is commensurate
with the dimensions of the upper jaw. And this is where we
sometimes get in trouble with you people. For in so doing,
we frequently invade an area which is rightfully the working
space of the tongue. As you no doubt know, the tongue is
a persistent and a powerful agent in the growth and development of the lower jaw, and no matter where we place the
arches or the teeth, the final position when we are all through
is going to be dictated by the space demands of the tongue.

With the average true prognathism, we have a massive lower jaw, the Dick Tracy chin, the Primo Carnera face, the acromegalic, heavy mandible; all these people have tremendous tongues. While we can section the jaw, we can take bone out, set them back, get them in normal relationship, then sit back; but beware. You had better get your records in the first six months because after that they frequently can tend to return as they were before. The tongue will insist on getting its space and you will be right back near where you started. When we do encroach on the field in which the tongue is most active, we sometimes impose an additional speech problem with which you must be patient and which we must understand and make allowances for.

The other area in which the orthodontist frequently runs afoul of you people is in the attempt to expand the maxilla. Rather massive appliances are occasionally placed in the area where the sibilant difficulties may already be rather pronounced. Even if you forget everything else I tell you, this is one area of absolute knowledge on your part where you can be insistent to a point where you can dominate the plan. There are a dozen other ways of expanding the maxilla without resorting to these large lingual screw jacks. And if you feel that this is going to be a prolonged impediment to your program, you should simply insist that the orthodontist change his appliance to something that is on the labial surface, or to something that is more diminutive, or to one that is removable for periods of training. And if he does not know how to do it, find an orthodontist that does know how to do it because I admit that these old-fashioned massive lingual arches are the easiest to use, but if it is going to invalidate two years of your speech training, it is a pretty stupid way to correct a dental malposition when you do have a choice.

Everyone says that in a malocclusion the easiest way to classify them is Doctor Angle's *one, two, and three*. In Class I, the relationship of the point of the mandible to the rest of the skeleton is normal. If we have the mandible diminutive in comparison to the maxilla, the Andy Gump kind of face, this is the Class II. Remember that this is not solely concerned with the teeth. This is the mandible. The teeth will have characteristic occlusal relationships in most instances but not necessarily so. The Class III is the "lantern jaw," in which the mandible is overdeveloped in relation to the maxilla. Conversely, you can have a variation of this in which you say the mandible can be normal and the maxilla underdeveloped, or you can say both jaws can be protrusive and we actually have bimaxillary protrusion. This is a common cleft palate hazard, in which a massive denture creates a bimaxillary protrusion in which even though the teeth are perfectly aligned, you have massive large teeth; the lips must make extreme effort to cover these teeth, if they can cover them when the whole denture is forward with relation to the rest of the anatomy.

All these things happen because most malocclusion of any severity is inherited or at least is genetic in its origin. We simply have a combination of incompatible genetic characteristics. And you have heard the old wife tale about "Well, you've got my mother's small jaws and my father's big teeth." That is not quite so, but for all practical purposes, it comes out about like this. Scientifically, of course, it is not true at all. Nevertheless, these things occur because the size of permanent teeth is immutable. It cannot be changed. By the fourth month of life, the dimensions of all permanent teeth are fixed but the size and dimensions of the bone are not. So we have a youngster with teeth intended for a six-foot-four frame. These teeth are determined in the fourth month of the child's life, but from there on, the child is subject to many misadventures in growth. If you were able to fulfill your inherited potential, you would end up six-foot-four, everything perfect, your teeth fit the bones, the bones came through with enough space to provide for what the Lord put in there, and hope they will make it. But this rarely happens. A youngster starts out, has colic, hits a plateau and recovers. He has a series of allergy crises and digestive upsets, each time dropping away from the optimum. From here on, the youngster is perfectly healthy, nothing ever goes wrong again. He can parallel this curve, but he can never return to it. So, what do we have? We have little Joe, five-foot-one, stuck with the teeth that were intended for a six-foot-four fellow, because the teeth cannot shrink; they cannot grow. They are there and the bone has to make the best of it.

This is why in the old days we used to broaden the jaw. We used to stretch the bone and then step back, and six months later it all went back. It looked just like it did the day we started. We now know that since we cannot grow bone, we must reduce the amount of dental material that is competing for space. This is why, in most severe orthodontic problems, extractions are necessary—extractions of permanent teeth. You cannot grow the bone, so you must reduce the amount of dental material until it is commensurate with the bone that is available.

I would like to get down specifically to areas that are the nitty-gritty part of our mutual problem. You can be very effective in dealing with orthodontic management difficulties because you have the position of a third person. You can be a neutral observer, allegedly. The children in your care, whether cleft or not, will depend on you, as will their parents, for guidance in anything pertaining to function of the mouth. If you can develop an understanding which helps you lead the youngster across some of the hard spots in his orthodontic treatment, it will be a great service not only to the orthodontist but also in letting the probably disturbed parent realize that there are little difficulties that accrue to the speech process during this time that may or may not be significant. It will be your job to decide which ones are significant and which ones are transitional or predicated simply on a temporary placement of a short-lived appliance which will produce no long-lasting difficulties.

How do we diagnose a case? We want you to understand our jargon for just a few of the principal items so that when you send a child to an orthodontist and you get a report back from him you at least know what he was trying to tell you.

The method of determining in what areas these extreme problems fall can only be adequately and competently done by the use of a head film which is called a *cephalograph*. This is not just a head film—you must realize that this is an oriented radiograph in which a head positioner immobilizes the head through ear positioners and a frontal fixation device so that this child's head can be returned to exactly the same position year after year after year. When we take a series of these cephalographs, with the head returned to the same position, we can then plot which part of the jaw is growing and which part is failing. We know the angle and the position of the teeth that are buried. We know the size of the teeth. We can determine the direction in which they are migrating, even though they have not erupted, and we know where we can rob Peter to pay Paul and this is the big secret. If we can steal a little space here and a little space there, we can very frequently fudge our way to a successful result, which we could never do if we did not know what the growth pattern is going to be.

If we project these growth lines and see over a period of time that this child is going to have a massive lower jaw, how disastrous it would be to take out the four permanent teeth too soon and end up with multiple spaces because the jaw finally did grow to what it seemed to have no inkling of being able to achieve earlier. So this is a cephalograph. From this is made a tracing. Since there are so many other shadows in this type of thing, a skilled technician makes a series of tracings from this. These are called *cephalograms*. By eliminating the undesirable landmarks in the film, you reduce it to the essence of what you are interested in—tooth position, growth center position—and by comparison, you can make linear studies with some validity and almost predict, in most cases, where you will be three years from now, four years from now, and five years from now. This is the prime diagnostic aid.

Then come dental casts. These are actual impressions poured in a plastic material which stands the abuse of students, and so forth, without fracturing the way plaster would. From this we can decide, roughly, whether it is a Class-I, -II, or -III malocclusion. We can tell the relation of tooth to tooth, but we cannot tell the position of the denture with relation to other skeletal landmarks. In other words, this whole denture could be very much forward and yet the cast would show normal, or it could be way back and you could have a witch's profile dished out. So dental casts are limited to only giving you a clue as to the position of tooth to tooth.

We also have oriented dental casts in which the cast is related to the orbital point, to the eye and the ear, and these are accurate. This gives you the dental picture related to other cranial landmarks. These are called *gnathometric casts*.

The other diagnostic aid which we depend on is scale photographs—clinical photographs, intraoral and extraoral. And, of course, the other routine dental films which show us little cavities and teeth that may not have a long, useful future, but, actually, don't help us much in determining the quality of the bone or the number of dental units that are going to make demands in our area.

Let us follow a case of an infant. The first time we know about it, we get a call and, as this is a simple case, they say, "We have an infant here with a cleft. You had better come and look at it." After a careful appraisal to assess the problem we then decide, Does this case merit a silastic palatal splint? Or, Is the case sufficiently severe so that we should consider a bone graft, and then support? Is the case likely to respond to routine, conservative orthodontic treatment and be allowed to go its way for five or six years? This initial determination can be the greatest single key factor, and I want you to write this down because this is the text for the day: Sustained orthodontic management is the primary and dominant factor in securing the optimum maxillofacial function—cosmetically, speechwise and occlusally. I am not sure that everyone understands what we mean by "occlusion." Occlusion simply means contact. But when we refer to occlusion, we refer to the manner in which the teeth meet, the manner in which they bite, and the position in which the jaw holds the lower teeth against the upper teeth. This is dental occlusion. Ideal occlusion is rare, but normal occlusion allows considerable variation. You can have irregular crowdings, such as I have in the lowers. This is not a deformity, this is not abnormal, and while it is not ideal, it still falls within the racial norm. You might have minor spaces. You might have little deviations and rotations and still have normal occlusion. I am sure you all understand this difference between normal and ideal. But when you have occlusion where the lower jaw comes up, the Class III, this exceeds the range we call normal. This is a malocclusion. If the lower jaw bites back like Andy Gump, a Class II, this is a malocclusion. If the jaws anteroposteriorly are normal, when they come together only two teeth touch at the back and you have the so-called open bite in front, this is a Class I malocclusion. Even though the anteroposterior position is right, there is a crossbite. This whole side is inside the lower. That is a Class I malocclusion.

The other area in which we share problems is the area of habits and this is a risky area in which to become involved with this group, I am afraid. But I will tell you the way that we have finally settled into our treatment of habit problems. Almost without exception, the most dreadful habit with which we have to contend is the deviate swallow, the tongue thruster, and this is right down your alley and as far as I am concerned this is your baby and you can sure have it. Nevertheless, this is one of the most disturbing influences we have in our treatment planning. It is impossible for us to make any determination of when, or by what means, or at what time, this habit might disappear spontaneously. We have one group of rather militant psychologists who throw up their hands in great horror if we install little cribs to restrain the tongue. Their slogan is that you are better off with a minor dental defect than a psychopathic child or an unhappy adolescent. Or, they claim the psychological repercussions of violently uprooting a habit with sharp barbs and a tongue rake are far more disastrous than any type of malocclusion would ever be. On the other hand, we have well-documented divergent groups which claim we should go ahead and treat the symptom. No one has ever shown a child to have suffered any but short-lived transitional repercussions from the use of any of the preventative barbarous-looking devices. If you do not know what a tongue crib looks like, we will pass this one around. Do not drop it. This is supposed to be placed on a child tomorrow morning, so you know that I use them. This is a benign gentle crib. There are no barbs on it because this is a seventeen-year-old girl with a tongue thrust. Every time her tongue goes forward, it will simply hit this little crib and will not squirt out between the teeth. Eventually, if she persists in driving against it, it will make the tip of her tongue sore. If this does not work, the next step is to put a couple of little sharpened barbs on there. Does this sound barbarous? That is ridiculous. You have at least twenty-eight sharp, hard teeth in your mouth. You bite your tongue occasionally but pretty soon your tongue learns to avoid being in the wrong place at the wrong time. Otherwise, your tongue would be mutilated in very short order. Hence, if your tongue can learn to dodge twenty-eight hard, ivory spikes that come together fourteen hundred times a day, it can certainly learn to avoid an uncomfortable position against a crib. We have all bitten our tongue and I am not sure that I show any psychological manifestations of having done this; maybe I do. But I will tell you, my tongue learned not to go back there for quite a while, and this is all we ask in this crib.

In addition, there is a more sophisticated and a much more costly device in which we have little mercury batteries that are buried into one of these plastic palates; we use a device like this with two little mercury batteries and a little transistor and two probes. Every time the tongue comes forward, it gets a real good electric jolt, and the eyes light up occasionally. But we are a little hesitant about using this because most youngsters have an awful lot of divergent metal in their mouth. They have silver fillings, gold fillings, different degrees and different types of alloy, and it is very possible that you can set up some galvanic electrolytic exchange with some irritability to the teeth. While this little battery palate is a great thing on paper, I have not had enough courage. I have made them up twice and I have lost my nerve at the last minute and did not place them on the child. But it is something that I might be tempted to use if I cannot lick the problem any other way. At least we know it is back there if we need it.

The other habits that are not quite so deadly, of course, are the tongue, the thumb, and the finger-sucking habits. We are not concerned with these particularly, unless they persist past the fifth birthday. So, it is pretty hard for us to get excited about a mother who brings a three-year-old child in and says, "I don't know what to do, the youngster has got his thumb in his mouth all the time." We say, "Very good. If it is still there in two years, come back and then we will consider it." But unless it is carried past the fifth year, any damage done usually is spontaneously resolved when the habit dies out. Fortunately, eighty percent of them disappear under social pressures the first year of school.

The attack on habits can become so involved that many orthodontists have within their complex—where two or three men work in one office—a speech therapist employed almost full time in tongue-thrust control. And in the East and in southern California, this is the routine thing. You just are not an orthodontist unless you have a tongue-control clinic in conjunction with your practice. It is a little hard for me to get quite this excited about it.

There are other habits such as lower lip biting and the ticks and twitches that go with strange occlusal patterns. Almost all adolescent girls go through a two-year period of biting their lower lip when they are contemplating something or other. And we cannot get worried about this. But this is a normal posture. Maybe it gives them the heavy lower lip, the sultry mouth, or whatever it is supposed to do. But, it seems just to be there. All adolescent girls bite their lower lip for a couple of years. And it does not seem to do much damage. It sometimes spaces the upper incisor teeth, but this readily goes back with a little restraining device and disappears. This is not of any concern to the speech people. We want you to know that we know about it and a lot of other strange habits, but they are not of mutual interest to us, and I am not going to spend a lot of time on them.

I am going to get back to the orthodontic management as the primary factor in securing the best potential, possible result for a cleft palate child. This means we must watch this youngster, decide very early which teeth have a prolonged normal expectancy and preserve these teeth. We must have them and having them is probably the key to the difference between a nice, simple uneventful case and a case in which we have a long series of minor crises and eventually a very poor result. If we can have real knowledge of which teeth are not going to be deformed and we can determine this radiographically, we will allow these teeth to usurp the space of teeth that are in the line of the cleft, which we now know are deformed and hence cannot have a useful future. In other words, we start sacrificing teeth very early. We do not have enough—and the word sacrifice is wrong. We start trading space very early by eliminating teeth. We have a limited amount of space; if you allow a misshapen tooth bud to continue to grow in the line of the cleft and use this space, it will misdirect, misplace, or steer other useful teeth into a malposed position and it can actually deform the shape and size of the roots and crown. But if we know that this is a useless tooth and eliminate it early, you then leave the space available to the teeth that are competing for this room with the hope that a good, well-formed, useful tooth will take this space and become an abutment for a prosthesis later or a candidate for movement to fill the space or for alignment by orthodontic treatment. This determination must be made very early, that is, the average child has seldom seen a dentist by the time this determination should be made. We suggest age five.

I think it is important if you are going to have an impact of any consequence on the orthodontist that you have a working knowledge of at least the names of various types of appliances. Do not call it a *dojigger* or *whatchacallit*. Look at the thing and identify it and if you are not sure, look it up and see if it comes close to something. If you do not hit it right on the nose, at least you will be close enough so that when you are talking to the dentist about it he will know what you have in mind and he will certainly be impressed in the fact that you took at least enough interest to call it by a name that does have some meaning to him.

In sequence, these are the ways in which appliances are used and these are the names.

A silastic supporting splint, a little so-called *magic-plate*, holds the parts in position and neutralizes the strain of the repaired lip to prevent the overlapping of the segments of the maxilla and the premaxilla. This is the first appliance with which any one of you will have any contact. You will not have much to do with this except you should know about it, and some parent will tell you that at one time or another their child had to wear this. Unless you are familiar with it, you might feel that they are dreaming this up—that no such thing exists. But it does exist. They are fairly new. They have been used for approximately seven years with considerable success in various parts of the country, and as the materials have improved, the effectiveness of the device has improved. It has now become almost a specific for certain types of unilateral clefts with uniform success.

The next device with which you may have some contact will be a little gadget called a *space maintainer* which is frequently placed by the family dentist to prevent drifting of teeth following the too-early loss of a primary tooth or even a permanent tooth. This is a simple device which should rarely, if ever, cause any complications in your field. It usually consists of a small screw or a little spring which simply holds the two remaining teeth on either side of the gap in a proper vertical position so that they do not tip in and steal the space that should be maintained for the late arrival that may not be due for four or five years. These are not an unmixed blessing, and for your own edification, if the child has a space deficiency in the jaw already, placing a space maintainer is a fruitless operation. It does not do a bit of good to hang on to half as much space as the tooth that eventually comes in there will need. In fact, if you are going to have to remove teeth, and almost all cleft palate children have to have two lower first bicuspids removed, this is the area where most space maintainers are placed. We may only need three millimeters of space but we cannot extract half a tooth on either side; we have to extract a whole tooth. A space maintainer will hold half a tooth for us, but without it we would not lose more than a whole space of a tooth and it is the whole tooth we take out, so a space maintainer that holds space in an arch that is already deficient in capacity for all the succeeding teeth is a waste of money and a waste of the child's and your time.

The next device commonly employed in this part of the country will be an *expansion plate*. When I talk about this, I am talking now specifically about cleft palate children, not the normal child. These plates are of several kinds. They have a little threaded segment in the center and a little wrench. With an intelligent parent, you can place one of these, let the parent take this wrench, or something like this, and they can crank this open one turn a week or a quarter of a turn every other day depending on how mobile the segments are. In this case, this is simply the split plate which, as you turn the jack screw, opens wider and moves the two sides out of crossbite, which is the thing we talked about before. And this, unfortunately, is going to be the worst thing in the world for conflict in your training program for several reasons. In order to hold the jack screw, it requires a rather substantial bulk at the palatine area, the sibilant area immediately lingual to the four incisor teeth. In addition, as the thing is cranked open, it exposes two parallel, or nearly parallel, edges with a slight taper at the bow, so as the tongue comes forward in routine movements, it encounters a rather uncomfortable crevice and actually gets pinched occasionally. There is no way that even the most skillful tongue operator can seal both the anterior and the posterior part of the palate to avoid escape through the split part of the device. Therefore, any assessments you make of a child's speech deficiencies or potential with this in place is an absolutely meaningless assessment. If you ever see one of these, remove it yourself or have the child or the parent remove it at least for twenty minutes before you make any judgment as to progress or lack of progress or potential for future retraining. This is the worst offender in your area, in all probability.

The next and more satisfactory way of expanding the palate is one that you may have heard about. It is called a *Porter-W*. There are permanent bands fastened on the posterior teeth. This goes into the palatal area and is put in under compression. Then, as it tries to relax, it expands and carries the two halves of the maxilla out with it. This still has the misfortune of encroaching in your area and, as it expands, it usually drops down and becomes a rather substantial hurdle to the facile movement of the tongue.

Consequently, a *maxillary lingual arch*, and this is actually called a *Mershon lingual arch*, with expansion springs, is a safer, more gentle and less hazardous way of doing it. You can see the very small gentle auxiliary springs and you can actually see where it has moved these teeth because the heavy body wire is where the teeth were when this was placed and the little gentle springs have moved it this distance over a period of probably eight to ten months. Elastic bands are used as an adjunct to the Mershon removable lingual; this is commonly used after most of the permanent teeth have arrived. This means you are getting into an area of some sensitivity on the part of the youngsters twelve and thirteen. So to a Mershon lingual arch can be added temporary cosmetic space fillers which can be changed periodically. As the space opens, you can add another one, and another one, and another one, so the youngster avoids the sensitivity of running around with a large toothless gap during this period of therapy. After we are past the active period, we can always put these things on a retaining device but there are just certain appliances that are amenable to carrying artificial teeth during the period of strenuous mechanotherapy.

In the maxilla, after the active stage has been completed, a device called a *Hawley retainer* is constructed. Some cleft palate patients wear a Hawley retainer all their lives. If there is adequate bony support, if there has never been stability, if they cannot do successful bone grafts to fill in the space, if the segments remain continually mobile, and if there is a persistent opening through the palate with escape, the patient usually wears a Hawley retaining plate for four to five years until he is old enough so that some permanent type of prosthetic device can be employed. On a Hawley retaining plate, we also can add small cosmetic units to carry the youngster psychologically.

When you reach a point where you cannot tolerate any type of conflict on the lingual side of the teeth in your plan of treatment, we resort to *labial arches*. This is all done in the vestibule, in the mucobuccal-fold area. There is absolutely no encroachment in the area of the tongue. This is a more fragile, a more delicate, type of appliance. It is a little more costly because it requires substantially more permanent work on the youngster. There is a *twin wire labial*, which is a very gentle, very effective labial expansion arch. And, just in passing, when you are dealing with these children, if any of these little attachments come loose, point out to them that they must not be discarded. We all the time hear, "Well, that piece of tin fell off the front and we just came back to get another one." This metal is platinum and it is very costly, but we do not use platinum to be fancy; we use platinum because we must. It is the one metal that can be maintained in the mouth for long periods of time with absolutely no risk of corrosion in mouth acids. It is not affected by the ingestion of any strongly acid or alkaline food or drugs. It is softer than the enamel of the tooth so when we place it, if anything is going to wear or scratch, the tooth is going to scratch our appliance rather than our appliance scratching the enamel of the tooth. The funny thing is that it does look like tin and when they throw them away, it is a low blow. Then, following the use of this type of expansion, we frequently have a tendency when appliances are taken off for some minor shifting, or new teeth arrive which require a little more space than we planned.

A device which will be the next thing you will run into is called a *Whitman elastic retainer*, and this is how it is made. The teeth are cut from the model, just so you know, and repositioned in an idealized form, even though they are a little irregular. Then, this device is made up. The back part, the clear part, is rigid, but the yellow part in front is slightly elastic, like gum rubber or latex. When this is forced back into the mouth with the irregular teeth, as the latex tries to relax, it carries the teeth into the idealized position until it exhausts the displaced rubber. The nice thing about this is that it can be removed readily by the patient and usually is. But it usually is used at ages fourteen and fifteen so that the youngsters take them out for parties, lovemaking, and stuff like this and I do not blame them. They are quite fragile and easily distorted and we do have to worry that sometimes after they have been bent a little bit, the youngster tries to put them back in, and of course, if they are warped, it warps the teeth into an undesirable position. This is why we actually endorse their removal for lovemaking, because once they have been rolled on, they do not work well.

For minor tooth movements, the most commonly used, and probably one of the appliances with which you will have the most frequent association, is called the *labial-lingual technique*. This is an appliance in which you have a fixed arch inside to move the teeth out and a removable arch on the labial side, and you can feel the tension here, to avoid letting the teeth go too far. In other words, it acts like a template; the inner arch moves out until it hits the fence and then it stops. This is the type of appliance, for instance, that in our office, we put on youngsters that are going away to Maine for three or four months in the summer or going to Culver for a semester. This type of appliance will work over a long period of time with very little risk—and very little danger—and this is the most common of all the cleft palate cemented appliances. Either the lingual part or the labial part can be readily removed so you do not interfere with the treatment. If you want the lingual part out for five months to try something, the orthodontist can slip the lingual part off and the labial part goes right on working, or vice versa.

There is a more sophisticated appliance that gives you control in two or three dimensions. In other words, with a wire lying against the teeth, you can push them in, you can pull them back, but you certainly cannot rotate them. Neither can you torque them unless you can get hold of them. So with a wire leaning against them, you are restricted. The more sophisticated appliances are called *multiband* and these are the ones when you see the kids running around town with a mouth full of railroad tracks. They are probably the most effective, and there is this about it: That since each tooth is protected with a sealed platinum sheath, the danger of damage to the enamel or caries is minimized because the springs ride against a protective shield and never touch the tooth itself. They are quite costly to put on because they have to be fitted to each tooth; they have to be removed periodically for prophylaxis and operator check, but they are by far the most efficient from a mechanical standpoint.

There are three subdivisions of the multiband and you might as well hear about them because this is where we run into the problem of emotionally polarized disciples in treatment philosophies. If you can imagine grown men coming to blows over whether or not you put a round wire or a rectangular wire through the bracket, this is entirely the basis of the greatest split in orthodontic philosophy in the world. This, and this alone, has blown universities apart as far as their graduate orthodontic training is concerned. If you use a round wire it is a *Johnson*, actually it is a *Johnson twin wire;* this is the way you will hear it and you will hear men beat their chest and say, "I'm a Johnson twin wire man," and you are supposed to fall on your face and be duly impressed. There is a *Begg;* this is called a *Begg light wire technique.* Doctor Begg is an Australian; it is also called the *Kangaroo technique.* It is a very, very effective technique, one of the very best and how this man without any formal training ever came up with this thing down in the backwoods of Australia we do not know, but almost every orthodontic department in the United States now is trying to get him to give seminars on this technique. This is very resilient and resembles the Johnson. The Begg can use both round and rectangular wires.

Then, the real fanatics favor the *Angle edgewise mechanism.* Angle does not mean two lines that converge. Angle is a man's name; he is the patron saint of all orthodontists— Edward H. Angle. And, of course, he is spinning in his grave because he taught that the Lord gave you thirty-two teeth and who are you to impose a better type of architecture by eliminating some permanent teeth in order to get a good occlusion. I have been doing nothing but advocating removal of teeth for twenty-five years and I am sure Angle has not had a good day's rest since. But he devised a rectangular wire and it is called *edgewise arch* and it is a good one. Improperly used it can be brutal, but it can also give the finest degree of control. Do not be impressed because somebody says, "I never use anything but Angle edgewise." This is like going to a doctor who says I treat everything with iodine. A well-trained orthodontist will use all these techniques, selecting the one which is the least cumbersome and is still effective enough to cure this particular anomaly. The rather slavish adherence to one tiny subdivision of the technique is sort of asinine from my point of view, but there are those who take issue.

We said that we expand the maxilla in a cleft palate child as far as we feel it can potentially maintain. In other words, there is no point in overexpanding because when you let go, the muscles, especially the buccinator, will collapse it back to a point of stability and the secret is mainly that the position of anterior teeth is determined by the backward restraint of the orbicularis oris group of muscles which are attached eventually to the median raphe at the back so you have a closed circle. This has a parachute-like action against the teeth. This is why, when you swallow, you must close your lips to swallow, because when you swallow, the tongue presses forward against the teeth. This forward thrust is neutralized by the backward pull of the orbicularis oris group and you end up in a position of equilibrium.

If, for some reason, we lose the backward pull of this curtain of the lips (and at Children's Hospital, for instance, we have youngsters where the lips have beeen burned and we have lost it), even though this child had a normal occlusion, very shortly all the anterior teeth go horizontal. They become procumbent because the tongue then becomes dominant, the teeth fan forward in an effort to escape, and it takes very little pressure to move a tooth. You could move a tooth with a hair if you could control the hair. The weight of a quarter would move a tooth all over the mouth. It will not move the jaw, but when we need this, we are talking about pounds— this is orthopedic-type movement. But as far as the tooth migrating through the bone is concerned, we can move it with the weight of a quarter or anything that exceeds blood pressure locally.

Thus, the final position of all teeth will be determined by the backward pull of the lip muscles as opposed by the forward thrust and the space demands of the tongue, and no matter where I put them, their final position will be a position of equilibrium, wherever that may be. If you have tense, hard lips, teeth will be retracted; they will all be in. They will be flat with a hard lip line. Trumpet players usually have this. If you have flaccid, atonic lips, if you have a posture where your mouth remains open, if you are a mouth breather, the teeth will tend to move forward due to this lack of restraint, and they will take a more procumbent position. These two positions can both be within the range of normalcy, but they can also exceed that range; this is what decides the axial position of the anterior teeth, particularly. That position is a position of neutrality between the forward thrust of the tongue and the backward action of the lips. Therefore, you must not overexpand the maxilla to the point where you place these muscles under tension, otherwise it will collapse immediately.

Once we have succeeded in getting the optimum amount of growth in the maxilla on a cleft child, we then turn to the problem of how to make the mandible fit this deficient maxilla. The most common thing is to remove a few permanent teeth and simply retract the teeth back. This can be done in several ways. However, if you have mandibular overgrowth, a Class-III tendency superimposed on a deficient maxilla, you then have an exaggerated disproportion which exceeds the possibility of management under conservative orthodontic treatment. This, then, requires a combination of orthodontic treatment plus a mandibular resection, and in our sessions at Children's Hospital, the question comes up time and time again of whether this is severe enough to justify doing a resection in the mandible in order to get it back to where it fits the maxilla. This is not a thing that you undertake lightly. This is a serious, rather major surgical consideration, and sort of a line of last resort. It is a prepared position to which you retreat only under the most severe of circumstances, but we have to be able to do it.

The case must be analyzed so that when we do cut a piece out of the mandible and carry it back, there is a position of stability which can be wired up and treated like a broken jaw until the bone fills in where you threw away the pieces on each side. Thus, we frequently have to position the teeth mechanically with artificial or orthodontic means to a preconceived pattern of stability; then it is cut; then it is wired back into position and heals in the new position. This determination of how much to take out, how much bone on one side and how much bone of the other and where the position of stability will be falls to the orthodontist and is done in conjunction with cephalometric films.

This is a Class III. I am sure that you can all see that the lower jaw is half an inch too far out. We do not make sample cuts on the youngster and say, "Whoops! Too much!" We do it on models, first, and then hope that it will work. We have an articulator in which models of the upper and lower jaw are set up and then we slowly grind away on the model, not the child, until we find that if we take this much out on the right side and one tooth plus this much bone on the other side, then this front section, which is now completely detached on both sides, can be brought back here, the two sides brought in, and then, when it is closed, you have normal occlusion. This is fine on the model, but the surgeon says, "How do we do this out there?" We then put the pieces back to their original position on the model and we make little steel, copper, or plastic templates, like this, and clearly mark them, so that even the surgeons cannot make any mistakes. This says "right" and this says "left," and the average surgeon can tell the difference between right and left. These are taken right into the operating room; after a flap has been laid back, placed against the bone, and a little line made with a dental drill on each side so they know they are getting exactly the right amount out, that section is cut out and thrown in the wastebasket. The jaw is then wired back up and you have an overdeveloped mandible that has been reduced surgically until it is compatible with the maxilla. And that is how this determination is made. That is called *osteoplasty* or *mandibular resection*, depending on what part of the country you come from. It is even called *osteotomy*. The three common sites of the cut, because it is something you hear about and talk about so you might as well be accurate—the most common site of the cut is just below the coronoid notch in the ascending ramus and this can be slid forward to overcome a micrognathia, or it can be slid back to overcome a severe Class III or prognathic mandible.

The second method or position of cut is a vertical cut through the ascending ramus and the face can be opened up and a piece of rib placed in there to advance the mandible, or an extra slice can be dropped out which will let the mandible be retracted. This is a vertical cut through the ascending ramus. The third method is actually to take a piece out just like we did here, for the determination, right through the body of the mandible, and this is simply called a *body section.*

In cases of extreme micrognathia where the lower jaw is too small and cosmetically undesirable, but functionally adequate, we can slide this forward after making a cut through the ramus, but frequently we lack the little mentle button, here; the jaw is still diminutive in its other dimensions so that you have a properly positioned baby chin on an adult face and this leaves something to be desired. So a simple adjunct to this, cosmetically, for these micrognathic children, is to make a small nick under the shadow line of the chin, and insert a little disc of cartilage. It can come from a bank; it does not have to be autogenous; it can be about the size of a quarter and any thickness and slipped in there. This gives a cute little button, sort of a "Hedy Lamarr" thing there and the nicest thing about it, is that it gives a semblance of character whether you have any or not, and this, after all, is what people judge you by and it solves a lot of problems. You know, if you look like a bulldog, you never have to prove that you are really a rabbit at heart; if you set the hands at twelve you are obliged to strike twelve times—that is the way it works. And so, if we give these youngsters the appearance of competence, if we give them the appearance of adequate competitive equipment, they will assume that they are adequate and competitive, and it is just that simple.

The other type of device is the type of splint that is put on after a section through the mandible. It is dropped on, tied with a button and then little rubber bands or chrome ligatures go to the upper jaw, and it is treated just like a broken jaw, like a jaw fractured in an automobile accident. It is held there and the patient lives on a liquid diet until you get some fusion between the two segments. It must have a stable position, a predetermined position to go to, because if there is mobility, you frequently get a fibrous union and a frail joint and then you never have a good functional result. This is why the preliminary treatment is so essential if you are going to have a mandibular sectioning. Especially with the cleft palate child, where the upper arch is usually not too stable, you must take advantage of every possible point of fixation in order to immobilize the broken segment below.

Now in summation, the orthodontist in the cleft palate team performs the following tasks:

(1) Preparation of diagnostic aids and records.
(2) Roentgenograms—dental, lateral jaw, cephalometric, profile, posteroanterior, and tracings of cephalograms.
(3) Casts and photographs, face masks, stents to prevent postoperative lip tightening.
(4) Orthodontic treatment—preoperative, postoperative, especially after surgery, and preparatory to insertion of prosthetic appliances.
(5) Determination of dentofacial growth status in relation to plastic surgery, orthodontics, and prosthetics.
(6) Correction of malocclusion.

Orthodontic therapy in cleft palate patients does not follow the same pattern as in children with sound palates and lips. Frequent limited amounts of orthodontic treatment are required over an extended period of time. There are latent periods in which the orthodontist must wait for certain teeth to erupt, for surgical intervention to be completed, for prosthetic appliances to be constructed, and for general growth and maturation of the patient to occur.

After all diagnostic aids, such as dental roentgenograms, photographs, impressions for casts, and cephalometric roentgenograms, are obtained, the orthodontist can cooperate in deciding when, in what order, and how much each specialty can do for the patient.

Chapter 10

THE ROLE OF MEDICAL
SOCIAL WORK

JUDITH BENSKY

MY GENERAL PLAN of presentation is that I will first discuss the generic descriptions, introduction, ideas, and techniques of social work in general; hopefully, this will prepare you for social workers you would meet, as much as to understand the particular specialty I have been engaged in for some time. Then we will talk about medical social work in particular, eventually discussing cleft palate work in particular, and I am going to indulge myself. I will describe a little of what we have worked with at Children's Hospital, since the rest of your team approach has been very largely from the hospital. Before I take up the case discussions, I would like to talk about what I think would be the nice thing to do—the ideal, the better thing, what I would like to see accomplished.

It is always good to have a definition of terms. You are lucky. To a large extent you can explain precisely what therapy is. To be sure, everybody talks, everybody is interested in hearing other people and in understanding them, but you have a definite scientific skill. I must admit that social service is an applied science. It takes a bit of this and a bit of that, and a bit of the other thing and adds its own particular quality, but everybody wants to get into the act. What is social work? It depends upon who you are. It is a long time since anybody who gave a Christmas turkey to a so-called "poor family" thought he was doing social work. Maybe for that time he was. We like to think of ourselves—everybody has a bias for himself, of course—as a helping profession. We do not so much do things to people until we find ourselves forced to do it, as we hopefully help them to help themselves. We also, and especially in medical social work, are a helping profession to the other professions. I think that is as important a part of our function as our own casework or group-work relationships. I think we are a profession. I think we are growing. But to a certain extent, we meet Flexner's criteria; we have a basic amount of transmissible knowledge, a concern for clients, and an interest in social program and policy.

I touched recently, just a little, on the history of social work. Certainly it goes back to biblical times. When one was asked to leave the corners of the field clean for the gleaners, to do justice, to have mercy for the fatherless and the poor, it was as a part of the Judeo-Christian ethic which is hopefully still a part of our present-day society. In other lands, in other religious cultures and civilizations, the plight of the poor has always been with us. Our only difference now is that I think we interpret the poor in a different way; as being not only poor in money, the poor in housing, the poor in food, but the poor in spirit, the poor in experience, the poor in ability to control, to help themselves to live a full, flourishing life. In our own country, I think much of our social work now is based on the Elizabethan Poor Laws with the use of residence and the use of taxes for care—as well as purely charitable donations. With the industrial revolution, with the change in philosophy; with the great revolutions, of which ours was the first; with the French Revolution and the many others, there came to be a rise in the feeling of the importance of the individual. Slavery and serfdom became no longer acceptable as a means of living nor as a part of the social structure. Helping people to be independent, to do for themselves, to be contributors to the society, I think, was one of the real bases for the beginning rise in social work.

Social work, as we know it, really dates back not much less earlier than the beginning of the twentieth century. The Charity Organization Society of New York started having courses to teach people how to be friendly visitors about 1898, and that course eventually ended up in the old New York School which is now a part of Columbia University. Again, with the political-social revolutions and the industrial revolutions there came a rise in the theory of the ability to rise—the right to make the most of oneself, the right to be flexible and to be important to oneself. But, very largely until the 1930's, the emphasis of social work, except in one field, was very largely on helping the poor. The depression changed all that because we all were poor. The basis of the structure in which we all thought we were going to live, on which we had legislation, on which we had program, was cut out from under us. Previously, financial crises had affected only the people who were already poor. The white collar, the entrepreneurs, and the managerial class might have had less but never were in danger.

The depression, in becoming a great leveler, changed the impetus and the focus of social work, as I said, except in one instance. That, oddly enough, was medical social work. In 1905, at Massachusetts General Hospital, Doctor Richard Cabot asked Mary Richmond to help him help his patients. Though the way we do things through our structure, and our theories, have changed since that time, essentially medical social work has the same desire—the restoration of health in all its aspects, and the attempt to help other medical and other professions in arranging that restoration of health. Mind you, that does not mean I think social work which does not handle money as such is holier than social work that does. Money is an important medium of exchange including exchange of concern as well as of goods. In dealing in other aspects, both of general social work and of medical social work, money is important.

Another thing happened as far as the depression was concerned. Social work then went beyond the voluntary agency which was giving the equivalent of the Christmas basket to the poor and which supplemented very heavily the old Elizabethan Poor Law rates and became changed to this extent.

The voluntary agencies no longer were able to come close to handling the flood of need for assistance in the form of money. We had, therefore, the enormous changes in the public agencies as we now know them. The Emergency Relief Administration ended up as our present social services, our Social Security, our present Department of Social Services. In terms of the money spent, what is spent through local, state, and federal funds is so much greater than any voluntary agency that the entire focus of social work and the entire responsibility of social work has changed.

It has changed in another way. Not only is it responsible for the welfare of the people whom it hopes to help but it has begun to feel that it is responsible for aiding the community to make proper planning for the people whom it affects. That is a far, far cry from Lady Bountiful who went out to leave a warm shirt and a load of coal and got herself a very warm feeling of having been so nice.

One should bring oneself to a situation—people are not to be treated as robots—but one should realize that you have a definite function and that the other person has the right to deny you. You do not have a right to impose yourself upon him.

In the last ten years, there has been another ground swell of change. Even during the worst of the depression, for the large part, social work was considered a middle-class activity done on an assistance basis to the poor. After the depression, when voluntary agencies sought other ways of being useful, it was used as a casework technique on the middle class, but there was not much interaction. All of us who read the papers or who have lived through this city last year must agree that the action and change of the community in what social work is expected to do is coming up from the poorer class to the middle class, as much as from the middle class to the poor. Part of this is reflected, as I will talk later, in the change in the use of personnel in social service agencies.

In the long run, in the great goal, social work has emphasized the ability to allow the individual to meet his needs and the needs of his family, and the group and the community to meet their best needs, to be able to use their own abilities to the fullest extent. We have a new or newer emphasis, although some of this has always been present. I think that as I see legislation, conferences, and other workshops, the emphasis now is getting to be increasingly on the abolition of poverty itself.

Since you are from both metropolitan and rural areas, you are accustomed to different ways and different places where social work is. In your smaller areas, on the whole, the people you come in contact with are people who have a legal connection such as the Department of Social Welfare, the courts, or the Public Health Department. In almost every state now there is an agency concerned with public assistance for people whose income is inadequate, for one reason or another, to meet the ordinary needs of life. Those standards vary from place to place. We may all be Americans, but we do not have American standards of welfare or living throughout this country. It is not necessarily just the South of which this is true. We delude ourselves when we feel that if one lives up North, everything is going to be lovely. It is not true. In Michigan, in Oakland County until two years ago, people on assistance had no money. Just imagine trying to arrange medical care for people who did not have bus fare. They had vouchers. The vouchers were for the clothing someone else thought they should have; for the food someone else thought they should cook. The assumption was that if you were needy, you were also stupid. What is more, you should be so extremely grateful for the ability to breathe that you should not question what you were given. That was not the South and that was not a poor state—that was Oakland County. Right now, in this state, there have been mergers of relief agencies, all the county agencies, into one state agency. It does mean that to a certain extent within this state, there are essentially basic levels beyond which a family should not go. In the metropolitan areas, the problem is that the cost of living is higher. There, the standards of assistance depend as much on what the county is willing to add to the state and federal grants as on anything else. To a certain extent that is fine. There should be some flexibility.

In the Department of Social Services now, there is general relief, which is different from categorical relief. General relief means a man who has just gotten burned out of his house and is without a job right now or the woman whose husband has left her and has nothing to live on right now. In our state there is a residence requirement. At the moment, in the Supreme Court, there is an appeal from a Connecticut court which has upset residence requirements on the basis that under the Constitution, people are entitled to travel between states and so are entitled to aid wherever they are. Up to now that has not worked that way. At the Hospital, for instance, we have a hydrocephalic baby who is very difficult to care for at home. The family has been here about three months. The State Hospital would take him, but it has an enormous waiting list. Nursing homes cost seven dollars a day. The county will not help, cannot help by law, because the parents have not been in the state for a year. It is those binds that are frustrating.

In the State Department, there are Children's Divisions in all counties now. If you have been reading, as many of us have, about battered children, that Division now is given the responsibility of initially dealing with these children. Children's Division also does child placement and some neglect work. They have a close contact with the Aid-to-Dependent-Children Division. With children in the legal sense, too, there are the courts, the Juvenile Court, and Divisions of the Probate Court.

There is a very large and useful division that works in the State Department of Health. I do not know what this state would do with cleft palate children without the help of the Michigan Crippled Children's Commission. Under Act 158, families are entitled to ask for and receive, depending upon their income and their ability, the care they need to make all crippled children as whole again as may be. When

you think of cleft palate, you think of orthodontia, prosthodontia, endodontia, oral surgery, and all the "dontias," of
plastic surgery, of visits to clinics, and of x-rays. Families that
are not able to assume that medical expense may be helped
by that Commission. This does not mean that people who
need help of the Crippled Children's Commission need to be
indigent or eligible for assistance of any kind—that is not
true. They need only to be unable to meet those medical needs
that are necessary because of the diagnosis. I can conceive,
and I am sure you can, too, of a family that makes ten thousand dollars a year and cannot handle plastic surgery and orthodontia, especially if there are other debts.

I would like to tell you a little about how one applies for
Crippled Children's Commission so that as you meet your
students whom you think may need this help, you will know
how to direct them. Parents or legal guardians may apply
either at the county Department of Health or, here in Detroit, if they are coming to a hospital, at the Michigan Bank
Building. Their application first must be a physician's certifi-
cate on which is the name of the patient, his address, his
guardian, his parents, history of his condition, the diagnosis,
and the statement that he needs to be cared for. It must be
signed not by any physician, but by a specialist in cleft palate
work. So many families have suffered so much with children
not given adequate care when they needed it, with the optimum of recovery less because it was started too late or not
kept up intensively enough, that I have made myself a one-
woman crusade to let people know that these facilities are
here; not only are they here, but it is in the interest of the
community that they be used. The community needs people
who are as well able to participate as possible. In the long
run, it is a lot cheaper to help a child become normal, or nearly
normal, so as to be able to support himself than to have less
participation from someone who has not been completely
restored.

There are, then, many private agencies which also touch
upon the lives of the children who are handicapped. There

are also children whose own families are inadequate to meet their needs, either through neglect, dependency, abuse, desertion, illness, or mental illness. In Wayne County, Catholic children are placed by the Catholic agency, Protestant children by the Children's Aid, Jewish children by the Jewish agency, and now there is a beginning of some foster home placements in the Department of Social Services and some by the Juvenile Court. In the rest of the state, Michigan Children's Institute and Michigan Children's Aid Society, which acts as a nonsectarian agency, are helpful in these cases. They are particularly helpful with children such as those with cleft palate, since because they are not as limited by law or by paper work, they are likely to be more flexible.

Then you have families who may need family casework beyond the relatively short-term contacts that the medical social worker may be able to offer. Those families can be handled by many of the family agencies of which there are a good many throughout the state. However, for the child or the mother and father who need intensive psychiatric care, unless there is enough money to pay private psychologists and psychiatrists, there is no private agency. They again have to go to a public agency under the Department of Mental Health, such as the Child Guidance Clinic or the mental health clinics. Their great need is not only community mental health but real emergency mental health facilities. Under the new Act, some of the counties are trying to do and have done much better than they once did.

In the agencies, social workers have different functions. In the hospitals, one is not so much responsible to a social work supervisor as to a doctor, who may not know what you are doing. The private agencies are run and supervised by social workers with social work attitudes, processes, and goals. In the public agencies, social work supervision is political and I do not mean that in any demeaning sense of the word at all. If you need to have a high-level policy determination on assistance, you are not likely to get it from a social worker in a public agency. Of course, the courts, as you know, are run by elected personnel and are under Civil Service for the social workers, the referees, and all other personnel. In public health, we have more social work consultants who work with the medical and nursing staff. Here I would like to put in a plug for the wonderful work many visiting nurses and public health nurses do with cleft palate children.

Funds in the public agencies obviously are provided by taxes and come through the legislature. In the private agencies, they come from many places. They can come from grants, endowments, and United Community Services. Sometimes public grants, such as from federal projects, are given to private agencies. Hospitals, of course, have insurance fees and fees from state and county given for services and not for budget.

Social workers will be found under many guises. They are in the family agencies, the children's agencies, and those dealing with general relief or categorical relief for people who meet certain definite standards and needs, such as Aid to Dependent Children, Aid to the Disabled, Aid to the Aged, and Aid to the Blind. Social Security, which is insurance and not a grant of assistance, has social work consultants with very few social workers, so that the family who, let us say, gets $240 from ADC has a social worker; the family who gets $240 in Social Security Survivors Insurance may have the same problems or more but does not have a social worker unless help is gotten from a private agency. Social workers are used in the psychiatric facilities such as the mental hospitals, the mental health clinics, the child guidance clinics, in public health, in corrections and the courts, as well as in the prisons. One important use for social workers is in group work such as the Y's, the settlement houses, and recreation. In community planning and in community organization, there is getting to be more and more interest in social workers, also.

I wonder how many of you have frequent contact with one of the very important divisions of social work—for the schools. Who are the social workers? What can you expect? Historically they vary, and, at present they vary. Historically there was no definite basis; anyone who did something that was called social work was called a social worker. In the Depression, a great many people who had very little educational background and no formal training became social workers because they did what social work was done in that agency. Then the trend was to more formal training as there is in every profession and, I am sure, in yours. After the Depression, the newer people who were coming in were supposed to have at least bachelor's degrees. The great push was on for postgraduate training. That training had been available since the beginning of the century, but it has become a two-year program leading to the Master of Social Work degree. In addition, there has been another step available through the National Association of Social Workers, which is a professional organization for MSWs in the Academy of Certified Social Workers, which requires two years of gradute work plus two years of supervision under someone who is already an Academy member. There has been a great drive, as in speech therapy, to have registered workers meeting legal needs and legal qualifications. In some states, there is legislation now pending or already enacted, providing for registered social workers. I hope that helps the clients; sometimes I think that just helps our own opinion of ourselves. More and more there have been some openings for doctoral programs.

In medical social work, there has begun to be a blend with the medical social worker between the Master of Social Work and the Master of Public Health. However, we are meeting personnel problems these days because of the enormous pressure for manpower which the graduate schools cannot begin to satisfy and because of the greater number of social agencies, social funds, social desires, and social legislation. The one hundred thousand people who are social workers with some training are almost a drop in the bucket. With the new poverty programs there has been an attempt not only to have people help themselves but to govern helping themselves.

There is also the use of nonprofessional and indigenous

personnel. Nonprofessionals are supposedly people who have no formal training for the work they are doing. Indigenous personnel are people who are poor and who are given the opportunity to help or to work in some of the poverty programs. In other words, the trend is to give jobs in the program. What this has meant I am not quite sure and do not think anyone knows as yet, but to a certain extent what it has meant is the breakdown into levels of competence of jobs that are to be done. In our own agency, for instance, you do not need a Master of Social Work, necessarily, to bring a patient into Cardiology Clinic. You can follow up that appointment, call the mother, make another appointment and, if necessary, go out and see why she is not coming in. You do need a graduate person or person with training to find out why she has not come in three times in a row or why a mother with a child with a severe congenital heart condition is pretending it is not there, etc. To save the time of the highly trained person, you can break down some of these functions.

The other trend, and I think it is one I am sorry to see, is that with the proliferation of public health programs, public assistance programs, and public mental health programs and the demand for manpower, the graduate with the postgraduate degree, i.e. with the Master's degree, is beginning to be used more and more as an administrator. Is that not the problem in the schools, too? Often the good teacher or therapist is supposed to be not too good unless she becomes a supervisor over others, so losing her contact with the students. Many professions are meeting the same problem. Frankly, I am not quite sure that a person who can do skilled casework or group work is necessarily able to run an agency. This is another profession. I myself have been more and more respectful of the managerial know-how, in agencies of administration, as such, as a separate and highly honored profession.

Let us talk about why there are social workers. Perhaps we exist almost by default. Can you think of any other group that would be interested and willing to try to coordinate, to try to meet total needs, to bring people together?

If you start doing that, and some of you have done wonderful work on that, how much time is left for your own work? If the teacher in the regular class starts working with her child who does not say his /l/ right much of the time, when is she going to have time to teach reading? As a result, we are supposed to have a smattering of many things, and I hope a competence in some. I do not think there is now any other profession that envisages the entire family and its goals as part of the community and has the desire to help not just one person but the entire constellation of the family. The physician must be interested in his patient's disease; the teacher has her second-grade student, and does not have time or energy to work upon his elder brother or his younger sister who is not of school age. The public health nurse, again, does more of that but is not able to use all of the techniques that a family or group may need. For whatever it is worth, and we try, it seems to me that social work as of now is the only all-encompassing profession.

In our highly complicated society which does not bear promise of getting simplified at all, more and more I think people need a friend at court—an ombudsman, if you like; an intervener, a liaison person, a coordinator—and that is why there is social service. That shows in our education. We take social welfare courses, courses in human behavior, human motivation, courses in group work, courses in community organization, and courses in social administration, as well. The "basic eight," as we have called them, are social casework, social group work, community organization, public welfare, social administration, social research, medical information, and psychiatric information. In casework studies we talk about social roles and interaction, the development of personality, the cultural factors in behavior, the client-worker communication, the differences in function and in goals of class differences and values. I am just hitting a few of the high spots. Others are the effect of stress in social behavior, learning theory and its relationship to therapy, the discussion of the action and interaction between the client and the worker, the client as an individual, and the family as a client.

Values for all social workers encompass the worth of the individual—his right and his duty to self realization. The purpose of social work is helping the individual not only to work with himself but with environmental aid and manipulation. It is as important to help a family to find a place to live and to find a school placement for a child as it is to work through the problems that Momma had with her mother so that she can be a good mother to her child. They are both important; they are different techniques. We try, I think, to have a fairly uniform feeling of sanctions, of what the community wants from us, and of what the community's goals are which it expects us to help.

The same basic knowledge that I have talked about is dealt with in the theory of human development, community facilities, and so forth. We also use the social sciences, but we change them; we change emphasis. The science of politics is the same in social work as political behavior in the courts and on the street; but in political science they are interested in discussing the pattern of political organization; in social work they are interested in using the democratic process to help the individual and the family. In psychology, psychologists are interested in measuring behavior and describing behavior. Social work has to know enough of psychology to know the consequences of behavior, the motivations, the mechanisms. In sociology, all sociologists are not social workers and social workers are not sociologists. They are interested in describing and understanding the mechanism of social organization; we are as interested in aiding to restore health to poor social organization, to social systems as a help to the individual and the family. Anthropology is interested in describing culture and history of culture factors; social work is interested in knowing the effect of culture patterns on the individual, the family, the community, and the different divisions in the community. In economics, surely we need to know enough about supply and demand. Banking crises affect us and the work we do, but what we are more interested in is the application of economics to the lives of the people with whom we deal.

Meanwhile, social service, like every other profession, has had swings and changes in the basic theories. We started with doing good to people. We then were strongly affected by the Freudian revolution. Training of social workers, to some extent or other, is based on that, because of the general teaching of the motivations of behavior with more or less connection with unconscious motives. But essentially, consideration of the role of the unconscious, the role of the unconscious motivations, and the role of behavior as based upon the development of the child into the adult is basic.

Then we went into a diagnostic period in which we were more interested in finding out what was wrong and in being able to make a proper diagnosis as much as anything else. It was the era of the long casework study when possibly there was long silence between the client and the worker and it was called dynamic passivity. Some people got well that way, but it was kind of tough. But we decided that we could not just be the listening post, and besides, we are not psychiatrists though some psychiatric social workers with training do psychotherapy. As you may know, in many other countries, psychotherapy is done by lay people and not by medical people. Most of us common garden-variety social workers need to know enough so that we can have some insight and try to give the patient or the client some, but one of the things we need to know is when we cannot step in. Otherwise, one can do a great deal of damage. We had a period of training in which the ego support, the ego ability to cope, was the important thing and that is still with us. We have talked a lot in the schools about the importance of roles, of what each of us expects we are to do, the psychodrama that each of us lives in our regular lives.

One of our most recent concerns is the role of crisis intervention, which is a long way from the dynamic passivity in which I was trained. Now the assumption is that not only is it necessary to give the patient or the client insight but it also is necessary to help him move. In helping him move, you may have to do the moving yourself. So instead of the greater status being given to the therapy, we are now swinging back somewhat to the actual definite manipulation of the environment for the aid and comfort of the client. My feeling, as I will talk about later, is that crisis intervention is an important theory for use with the cleft palate child.

For myself I cannot conceive that there is any family in which the birth of a cleft palate child is not a crisis, and I wonder whether we do not have a social duty to a family to offer whatever help is needed, on whatever basis at that time. It is not the same help because it is not the same family, the same child, or the same background. But the availability of help seems to me an essential factor in dealing with the total needs of the cleft palate child. As a result, our education has revolved around casework, group work, community organization, social planning, social research, etc.

We have one other method of training which is used in greater or less extent, I think, in all professions and that is internship of a kind. In social work, we call it field work. It is a practical experience in a social agency in which social problems are met under the close guidance and supervision of a person whose job it is to teach you what you are seeing in real life and not in the books. I will not say it is more important than the courses because you do not know what you are seeing without the background to see it with. It is an essential supplement because you do not know what you are learning until you see it in action. In all accredited social work schools, there are two years of field work. In many schools this means one year in a family agency because that takes in the entire family and many general problems and a second year in an agency of specialization such as a child guidance clinic or hospital.

On the other hand, we are beginning to blur the lines a little bit. One of the developments in social casework is the use of group techniques. I sometimes wonder whether we are using it entirely for the patient or whether we are using a group because we do not have time to do the individual, one-to-one relationship. You were telling me about eleven children in a speech therapy class; it was forced on you and not a matter of choice. On the other hand, we are interested more and more in the action and interaction of groups. One of the things I would like someday to see, for those families who need it is a group meeting of cleft palate parents. I almost said mothers. I think one of the real disadvantages of social work is that because of the father's work, and so forth, we deal too exclusively with women, though in the profession itself we have more and more men joining in as a social need and a social fulfillment.

I think we are rather prissy when we do not meet reality. One of the realities is the use of authority as a tool and part of casework technique, group-work technique or community-organization technique. We have come a long way from the age when the Romans had the right of life and death over their children, and there are instances where you have to make a choice between the needs of one person as against another in the family—as against the whole family, as against the community. If a child is being badly treated, it is wrong ethically and from a social work point of view professionally not to be involved. It is a dreadful phrase, is it not? There are ways of doing it properly. The one thing I think all of us, as people and social workers, need to be sure of is that authority should be called for—actually for the needs of the patient or the client.

In Children's Hospital, we are confronted, I regret to say, weekly—very nearly daily—with the battered child. The Battered Child Act is a relatively recent development in social legislation. Before then, the patient or family could sue a doctor or anyone else who complained. It is an indication of change in functions and goals of society that you as school people and I as a social worker, as well as nurses and doctors, are not only allowed to complain when there is a battered child but are under legal obligation to do so. You do not have to prove it. You need only have reasonable suspicion. You are not the judge and jury and the prosecutor. You must not feel that you are the person who has to have the complete evidence. I say this particularly because of the severe forces, the destructive forces, that are often set in motion when a defective child is born. It is your responsibility and your legal duty to see that a child is properly treated. I do not necessarily mean given the latest record, if he is a fifteen-year-old, but I mean adequate clothing. Malnutrition, a broken bone, a burn, and tying up a child is abuse. There is child neglect as well. The one thing that is difficult, still, and that is very difficult to prove in the courts is emotional neglect. If the bones are in one piece, the child is fed, he is clean and sent to school but he is called an idiot and a simpleton and told he will never grow up to be anything. He is thoroughly demoralized—I am afraid you cannot prove that, but you should be on the lookout for instances of child abuse—for your own protection, by the way, as well as the child's. Authority, like money, is a tool, and all tools are susceptible to the person who uses them and the purposes for which they are used.

Social workers keep records, but they vary. One of the reasons we keep records is that we are a social profession. We figure out that the next person who comes along needs to know what we know. You do to a certain extent, too. There are people who feel that they have done it and nobody else is to question them. One of the advantages, if you call it that, of being a helping profession is that we assume that everybody has a right to question us. It is also to the advantage of the client because the next person who comes along does not have to ask the same questions to get a picture of the family constellation. It is to the advantage of both the client and the social worker because the supervisor knows what is moving, how to help, how to point out changes, growths, backwards steps, and what we work with. In other words, the record to us is a crystallized client. There are different ways of recording. Sometimes we use very quick summaries when we do not have time for anything more extensive. Sometimes, when we are actually doing what amounts to therapy, we use a more prolonged summary. Sometimes we lean over backwards in not imposing our own feelings and our own diagnosis on the next person, but try to give enough of the situation and description of the family so that the next person can come, hopefully, to the same conclusion. We hope, also, that someday records will be used for research. We have ideas. We talk to each other as you do. I suppose in all professions, really evaluative, objective research has not yet been done as adequately as it should have been.

When I talk about records, I talk about supervision, and there again, more than in many professions, supervision has been a social work tool as much for the protection of the individual client as for the growth of the social worker. Like everybody else, some of us do more than we think we do, but the supervisor is also used in an attempt to see that one client is given the reasonable quality of attention that every other is and that things are not left undone that may be done. We conceive of ourselves as an evolving profession, that we ourselves grow as we deal with people, we ourselves grow as we learn more. One of the ways we grow is by having someone else sit down with us and evaluate and discuss what we are doing.

Certainly we sit down with the client and evaluate and discuss what he is doing. That, of course, is interviewing, which is an important part of social work. Lots of occupations use interviewing; lots of professions do. Any time people talk to each other there is interviewing, but hopefully social work techniques are such that interviewing becomes a meaningful process and something that will teach both us and the client what we are working for. Interviewing then brings us to the one thing that medical social work and other social workers are relied on to do, and that is history taking. Doctors take histories and should; a diagnosis can be very different if the history is adequate or inadequate, full or not full. Social diagnosis also depends upon history. The same situation, the same illness, the same learning disability has to be evaluated differently depending upon the situation of the entire family, the child's past history, the milieu in which he lives, and the different goals and views which he has. A history, then, should give a crystallized picture of social forces in a social situation in the family if you are doing medical social work. Social work history varies in degree, not so much in kind, because we are interested in the entire group. If you are doing a history on your student, you are interested in what his speech has been. I presume you are also interested to a certain extent in how his family speaks and what they mean for him. We are, or should be, interested in not only how they speak but how they feel, what other motives they have, and what other problems they have.

I have often discovered in history taking that what was brought to me as a situation is not the real problem. The woman who comes to ask for dental work for her cleft palate child may really be in a marital situation which badly needs aid right then and there. Or you may find that another child in this family has an emotional disorder which severely hampers the ability of the family to handle the illness of the child. So social work history is more embracing than any other I know of.

Our goals in casework involve a relationship with the individual and the ability to help him help himself. In some situations they can get along moderately well if there is just someone there who can be called on. You do not have to make a lot of movement; you do not have to make marvelous changes; you need not wave the flag and say, "Look what I did." But you can often help a family keep going.

The other roles are the manipulative ones I have talked about in which the environment is helped. Situations in which another agency is asked to give the help the child needs can be manipulative. I used to feel that that was a less worthy thing and that therapy and insight were far more valuable and more "statusful," if you like. I think that I have become more realistic in that my goals have become realistically limited. I think the manipulative function of social work is extremely important, there again, because no one is that interested in as much of it.

We also have a strong function in interpreting the needs

of the patient, of the family, and of the community to the people involved. If the child has an illness or a handicap and the doctor prescribes a certain treatment, parents may or may not be able to carry out that treatment for one reason or another. Maybe they cannot do it that way, maybe you have to take more time or do it elsewhere or interpret in a different way. In medical social work, it works the other way. Many times doctors and nurses and therapists use language that some people do not understand. A social work job is to interpret to the client what you want, why you want it and how it is done, in a way he can understand and accept, so he will cooperate with you. In doing this, I do not know that I can say that any social worker can put down a long list of things. You have to think with your background, your knowledge, and your hopes. In our case-work relationship, you can try various grades and levels of what you are hoping to accomplish, depending on your own abilities, on the social situation, and on the abilities of the family. There are people who can actually gain a great deal of insight and are able to move enough with their own skins so that they can help themselves help the situation. There are people who do things because you ask them to and they think you are a pretty nice person. They are the right things but they do not really know why and maybe you cannot help them. There are people whose attitudes you help change. When it comes to the relationship of parents to a defect in a child, those attitudes are enormously important, and the emotional forces that are set in motion are also enormously important.

Psychiatric social workers will work more on insight in the mental health clinics. All social workers should be able to do some—again depending upon the problems and the people. One of the techniques of social work is to aid in problem solving, in trying to communicate with the patient or his family so that they can see the aspects of a problem and see what they can do to meet it. One of the great advantages of social work is the knowledge of community resources. I talk about a manipulation, but I meant that as well, we are supposed to know what everybody else does. If you work in a hospital, you are supposed to know something about relief requirements. If you work in a relief agency, you should know something about child guidance clinic requirements. One of the things we do at the hospital is act as a resource person for people whom we never see, whose names we do not know. Despite the attempts to publicize what is available, so many people do not know. It is one of the reasons why I talked about the Crippled Children's Commission. Title resources vary. Part of the job of a reasonably good social worker is to know what is doing in all community facilities and all the things that people need to have and need to have done.

One of the things I did want to mention and talk about again is that except where the health and welfare of a helpless person is involved, and except where community standards are involved, a person has to refuse proffered aid. We would hate to live in a society in which we were moved around like pawns on a chess board or, rather, like checkers because chess at least has some personality involved. We need not feel that we are so wonderful or so easily accepted that there should be "hosannas" of joy whenever we approach. Many of us might feel personally upset because they do not know how wonderful I am—how much I want to help them. Help is a two-way street and unless you have to use authority, people have a right to refuse you; they have a right to decide that what you have to offer is not what they want at that time and time is an important factor. A family that may not accept something now may be willing to accept it later. That is part of social diagnosis. The obverse is also true. If you do not give a certain type of service now, they are not going to take it later. These are not mechanical people we move around; they are living human beings who, just because they happen to have a social worker walking in, do not lose any of their rights or their emotional privileges. Eventually, we hope that the amount of help we can give them in a family with any pretensions to help will work us out of a job. I have a sort of feeling that people who want to continue contact forever and are unwilling to give up a family are serving their own emotional needs and not the needs of the family. As social workers, we are expected to evaluate our own feelings in a situation as well as the client's.

One of the things that we do with other professions is to collaborate. As we are beginning to define different areas of necessary competence in our own work, I think one of the important things, particularly in illness, is collaboration. The one social worker should not feel entirely responsible for the entire situation or the entire family. There is room for the public health nurse, for example, where the social worker should not intrude. There is a function that the doctor has that is not the social worker's. One of the things we must be very careful about is that social workers do not make medical diagnoses. When there is a good relationship, a good collaboration, one profession knows where it starts to blend with the other one. For instance, in a child-placement situation the interpretation of illness is done by the medical social worker. But, the placement is handled by the placement agency. There may be a time when the hospital social worker should state because of this and this need, this is the kind of placement we would like to see, but as we give individuals the right to make their own decisions, you have to give other agencies and other learned professions the right to make theirs.

In some respects, the social worker does not enter in directly at all. In many of the public health situations, the social worker acts as a consultant. She can discuss what is needed in a situation. I went into a discussion on health services in which my role was not to say that Johnny Jones is coming to the medical clinic or Mary Smith is coming to the cleft palate clinic, but these are the facilities we have, these are what we should like to see for such and such a reason. We have had experiences in seeing how services are delivered and what this means to the people in need of them.

We may never see the person for whom this is meant, but we are useful in aiding and making a program and policy. Each of us has a sphere of competence and a division of knowledge—not hard and fast but focused.

One of the things I meant to say earlier is that not only are we aware of the fact that we can be refused, but we know it is not our business to be judgmental. More and more, social work has become less of a middle-class activity. We have to be careful that values and goals are not transferred to people who do not want them, do not need them and cannot use them. To be crass about it, illigitimacy is a middle-class disgrace and there are classes where it is a way of life. You cannot scold a woman for having children by different fathers if she does a good job of taking care of them. Everybody knows she does. There are people who do things that are most distasteful to you. That does not mean that you can write them off. You accept them where they are, as they are, and where they can go. As a social worker, they do not have to meet your requirements for where you are, as you are, and where you go. That does not mean that there are not community needs, goals, and standards. It is important that as a helper, the social worker accepts the client as, in himself, having some worthwhileness, no matter what his behavior is. That does not mean that you have to condone it or imitate it, but you must understand it.

We have already talked about the sources of funds and the special grants. One of the things we hope for is social work research. Each of us is trained in graduate work to do some of it. I think our tools for actual scientific evaluation are not yet perfected. It seems to me that one of the things you do that is most important is preventative as well as remedial, and how do you measure prevention? How do you measure intervening in a situation which then does not get worse. Yet in some way we have to learn how we measure and what we should do so that we can be more helpful and really do our work better.

Medical social work is a restoration to health, meaning

health more specifically than the restoration to good function which is the general goal of social work. Here, medical social work is under a certain difficulty and yet can be used as a help tool. We are an ancillary profession. It is not easy for professional people to find themselves under orders. It is not everyone who is comfortable in a medical social work situation. You may see a situation which is crying for help, but unless it is one of the things you have been given to do, you have to keep your hands off. At Children's Hospital, there are certain diagnoses in which social work is routinely invited. Those are the ones in which the particular illness is necessarily a family problem, such as rheumatic fever, diabetes, nephrosis, prematurity, cardiac involvements of certain kinds, malnutrition, failure to thrive, and of course, the battered child. You can see some other situations in which you feel you should, and could, and would intervene if you were permitted to, and let us face it, you are an ancillary profession, the doctor and nurse are in charge, and YOU ARE NOT! I do not think school people have quite the same thing, except that, of course, you are under administration.

One of the factors that we consider in medical social work is that illness is an important thing, but illness and the reaction to it do not change personality; they are only another function and another side of a personality that was already there. You can see the same illness in two different people with the same prognosis and have widely different reactions to each. In one family, a child is rejected because he is hydrocephalic or a mongoloid; another is tenderly cared for by the family. Illness, however, can be a particular kind of weapon. And I think you have seen that in children who have trouble in speech. Some of them have trouble because they cannot talk and some because they will not talk. There is a question as to whether they lose the psychic gain they have by not talking well, that is, the special place in the family, the special attention, the need not to grow up, the need not to be held accountable. However, I accept as a truism that all chronic illness and all defects are a stress on family life. I cannot imagine a normal human being smiling through it all. And if they do, then watch out. There is really a sick family, a terribly sick one, because they cannot bear to face themselves at all, and if they try, they are afraid they will shatter completely.

It is like the child who enjoys a hospital. Any family who just meets illness completely in its stride without any feeling needs to be helped. In dealing with illness, family strengths should be discovered as well as family weaknesses. Yes, illness is a stress. Yes, it is a function of personality which is preexisting. That does not mean there are no strengths or that you have to give strengths. A family may be able to recover from this stress and to come to a point which enables them to deal with this without a great deal of intervention. However, when illness with children is considered, the community goal is a restoration to health, and the community is as much your client as the individual or the family.

In medical social work, particularly within the agency, coordination is an important part of the medical social worker's function. The ability to coordinate, to get everything scheduled so that what is done applies to all facets of the illness is an important function of a good social worker. A patient is not only an illness. We had a patient in Renal Disease Clinic who was referred for speech therapy because part of the social worker's job in that clinic with chronically ill children is also to be interested in the development of the whole child. The child did not talk, the examination did not require his speaking; it was necessary to talk to the mother the first time and then the next time to get a picture of development. Sometimes you find that you need psychiatric help. Sometimes you find you need a dietician's help. People will smile and are afraid to say they do not know. For instance, we had one allergy patient who was not doing well. The mother knew that the child was not supposed to have wheat flour but did not know in how many forms wheat flour was found. She had to be helped to get the proper diet by a dietician. I learned she did not know by asking. Often social workers do the obvious. You would think anyone would know. You can never take for granted that anybody knows anything, including yourself. That child's asthma improved, not miraculously, but markedly, because a mother had been helped to get the kind of care she needed to be able to follow out the orders of the doctor properly.

One of the things we have to watch for as social workers in medical settings is that physical illness is acceptable, emotional illness is not. You will find loads of people worrying about the child who has cerebral palsy or muscular dystrophy, but this business of helping people help themselves—of learning to come to terms with what they have or not reacting in an unhappy way—that, nobody much is interested in. We feel that if you have given your all for the child who has a brace, we have done just fine because we have given them the brace. But the brace is only the top of the iceberg of his illness. The important thing is what he does with it, what it means to him, how he handles it, how his family handles it, how it is used or not used or misused.

One of the questions I have is whether physical illness is not too easily paid for by excessive dependency of the patient. As we talked earlier, we do not always know whether they do not want to give up the gain of having something wrong or are afraid that if whatever they have wrong is corrected they will have to meet life in a way they are afraid they cannot cope with. So it is easier to remain sick. I regret to say that schools are notorious in their unwillingness to accept physical illness and emotional handling of it and I do not see anybody disagreeing with me. A child who has asthma may be out a little bit more than the others, but the ordinary child with attendance difficulty is met with the attendance officer coming over and over and over again. I have known one child who managed to stay out of school most of the time till he was sixteen; but to keep an asthmatic child in school, there is a problem. An asthmatic child is gone two days one week and two weeks later, three days more. He is quietly on home teaching, which, of course, is completely calculated to increase his asthma. He needs a group experience.

Many agencies, I regret to say, are frightened by illness. As I said at the intervening period, we had a severely psychotic youngster who happend to have diabetes. We could not find a single mental hospital that was willing to handle diabetes. They were perfectly willing to handle severe acting-out psychoses, but the idea of sticking a needle with insulin into the child—well, you just cannot do that. People are afraid of physical illness. I do not know whether they fear it, whether it is kind of crossing your fingers, it should not happen to me, that you do when you meet a car with a flat tire on the expressway; or whether they know so little about it that it is something they shy away from. One of the reasons, I think, is because they assume a certain illness requires a certain reaction. That is just not true. Different families, different people, different situations, different results, and the function of the social worker is to individualize everything as much as possible.

I think I've covered briefly the function of the medical social worker. The other social worker that as therapists you are more likely to come in contact with is the school social worker, and a good half of you, or more, do have them. It depends on her training, your administration, your power structure, and what the schools prefer to have from her. There is one of your members who says her school social worker has acted as a perfectly marvelous community agent who works with children, works with families, refers them for added help, and is a source of ever-present help in time of trouble. And another of you said to me, "Why is a school social worker scared by everybody?" She feels that she limits herself purely to working at insight into the child. Possibly, that's what she thinks she is doing because essentially school social workers started when the emotional development of the child impaired the learning process. But my understanding is that there has been more and more a feeling that whenever the learning process is impeded by something in or out of the school, the school social worker should be involved, and the community agent takes that seriously. Your worker who takes refuge in just seeing the child and talking to nobody else takes the older point of view. I cannot feel, for myself, that their usefulness is limited to the discussion with the individual child, because if deep therapy is needed on that case, unless there is no other community resource such as a child guidance clinic, that is not strictly the province of the school social worker. It is important to have people who are able to work with the teacher, the child and the family so that the child comes back and has a reasonable way of getting along with people and a reasonable way of learning. School social workers do a fine job, by and large, in trying to understand more than many social workers in more than many disciplines the effect of illness on the entire situation of the child, and that is what they are supposed to be doing.

Now I am going to jump to Cleft Palate Clinic so that we can get to case studies, case histories, and some discussion. Cleft Palate Clinic at Children's right now is a team clinic. At Children's, the person in charge is a plastic surgeon. At Sinai in Detroit, the person in charge is an oral surgeon. At St. Lukes in New York, the person in charge is a resident in plastic surgery whose job it is to lead a teaching team. At Children's, we are not so much a teaching as a planning team and a treatment team. Social service has only recently been used in Cleft Palate except for financial referrals, and financial referrals require a certain kind of social history which is not as yet a complete one. Social service works with the speech therapist, who refers things that she thinks are needed for the cleft palate children. The studies I have are done, except for two, in conjunction with her. These are all people who have speech therapy of more or less degree at Children's Hospital and who are cleft palate patients, except for two. At Sinai, a social worker sees the child at the point of intake, before he is seen in Cleft Palate Clinic. The social history is done and then the social worker is called in on referral. The Cleft Palate Clinic plans for services and makes referral for social services. Usually, we have been called in for finances or for noncooperation.

I would like to discuss what I think would be a fine set-up, not only for the use of the speech therapist but let us say for my own satisfaction. I think that our speech therapist has felt that she has been able to use social service in enabling the family to make proper use of her services, in referring them for added services such as nursery school, school placement, evaluation of their school experience, and encouraging the parents to continue to explain what she is doing and to understand what the situation is and what her function is. She does very well at that, but sometimes there are parents who are disappointed. We have worked in consultation on discussing what realistic goals are for various of her patients. What would I like? I like to feel that cleft palate, as I said before, should be considered a crisis and social workers should automatically come in at the beginning, at the point of crisis, to establish availability, an open door, a feeling of a friend-at-court. Then, depending on the situation, there would be more or less involvement. I do not feel you can say everybody must be seen at such and such a time; everybody must have this or that; no. However, I would very much like to see periodic contacts again at the time when I think crises are likely to develop. The first contact I would like to see depends upon the feeding process; whether there is any difficulty with feeding the child—not only with feeding the child in order to avoid malnutrition but with feeding the child as an extremely important basic mother-child relationship. An infant learns to be accepted because it is fed—that is our first contact. The sucking reflex, the sucking experience, is an important part of most emotional growth. I would like to be able to assess at that time what the feelings of the parent are toward it. Sometimes I think that feeding difficulties take place because the mother is depressed and she does not have the psychic energy to go through the slow, time-consuming, painstaking business of feeding a cleft palate child. The feeding relationship often is shown in later emotional relationships

between mother and child and between child and the world
at large. A refusing world, a world that does not feed you,
that does not let you feel good and warm inside, is not a
world you are likely to trust. Infants feel who loves them and
who does not.

I would like to be around long enough to know whether
mothers talk to their children, whether they encourage their
cleft children to babble, or whether they feel they are just
not going to talk well, anyway, so why bother. I would like
to be around them long enough to discuss the need for speech,
for talking to children, whether there is a reply or not, for
enjoying the communication with them. In other words, I
would like to be around long enough to see whether the foun-
dations of emotional health are being laid in the cleft palate
child. Then, in the family that does that all right, I would
stay away for awhile. I would like to be around again two
and a half or three years later when they are really starting
to talk, when ordinary children are speaking in sentences and
able to communicate, for the same kind of evaluation of an
emotional situation with respect to communication and relationship to the world outside. Sometimes, cleft palate children, I think, are afraid to talk. They do not like to be laughed
at if their speech is different. They begin starting bad speech
patterns. I would like, then, to be able to say to the speech
therapist, "Will you evaluate this child to see whether you
can help him now?"

My next period of crisis, I think, is school age, with school
placement and school interpretation, to aid in working with
the family in working with the school. Sometimes the schools
can be impersonally cruel. Sometimes they can be extremely
helpful. But this is the first step into the outside world unless
the child previously has been in nursery school or there is a
speech therapist at the beginning of speech who must feel
that an important part of learning is the socialization of speech.

The next point of contact, I think, should be adolescence.
Again, I would like to see some research, since in adolescence
the body image is so important. I would like to know even

if the cleft palate and the cleft lip have been repaired and the speech is good, whether the adolescent still feels uncertain and is without confidence because he thinks of himself as he used to be. And in respect to that, there is vocational planning. Realistic vocational planning is rendered for those we cannot help completely in accepting themselves as being able to do anything that they would otherwise do with those who can.

I do not really think we ought to go on with them when they are grandmothers. I am perfectly willing to stop at that time. I am sure that Doctor Fischoff has talked to you about the guilt of parents who have defective children. He has talked to you about the mechanism of denial—refusal to admit that there is anything wrong. I would love to see some intensive, long-term work done purely for deciding whether we are really working on the right street. Are we saying that the mother feels guilty because we would feel guilty? Are we saying that the parents deny because we would deny? I have often felt that medicine's referral of the defective child who is mentally defective or highly physically defective for institutionalization is as much a function of their own fear that their own children might be that way as it is a need for the child himself. The mongoloid strikes fear into every heart. He does not need an institution. Mongoloids are nice, sweet kids—they just do not grow up much. But nine times out of ten most people who see a mongoloid say, "Put him away." Do their parents really feel that way or is it we who feel that way? Actually, maybe it is wonderful that, despite all of us, so many children turn out well.

One of the things I wonder about is the fact that there are parent associations for everything but cleft palate. This may not be important, but why is there not any parent association of cleft palate children? I would like to see some real research on the intelligence of children with cleft palate. Some of the studies without a great many members in it, not samples that are supposedly not too large, seem to show that there is a certain lessening of intellectual scores. Is that because the measurement does not allow for the difficulty in speech; is

it real? I do not know. But if it is true, that should be a
fact that you ought to bear in mind when you think of training the cleft palate child. Do we necessarily feel that social
adjustment must be bad? Anything we have done up to now
is inconclusive. I would like to see some—and there again
I go into the biological sciences—some idea why there are
more male cleft palate patients than female cleft palate patients. Is the school adjustment different for the cleft palate
child because he has more upper respiratory infection, more
ear infection, more likelihood of hearing loss? Is it enough
so that we ought to make special arrangements for them or
should we just go along the line that they are normal unless
proven otherwise? If we find more problems in families of
children with cleft palate, is it only because we really examine
them more closely or is it because they have them? If the
patient keeps early speech habits from before repair, is there
any carryover in emotional habits? Is the slow progress that
some children make in speech therapy because the parents
do not want to give up the defect or because the child does
not want to? Is it a justification for not doing things well?
Or is it a factor of other personality disorders that have nothing to do with the illness in itself or the handicap? And I just
said before that I would like to see more social research done
on real evaluation so that we know what we have done and
what we are doing.